# FUNDAMENTALS OF CLINICAL CHILD NEUROPSYCHOLOGY

BARBARA Z. NOVICK, Ph.D.

Departments of Psychiatry and Pediatrics,
Lenox Hill Hospital, New York, New York

MAUREEN M. ARNOLD, Ph.D.

Albert Einstein College of Medicine,
Department of Psychiatry,
Bronx, New York

1988

G&S

**Grune & Stratton**

An Imprint of the W. B. Saunders Company

**Harcourt Brace Jovanovich, Inc.**

*Philadelphia, San Diego, London, Toronto, Montreal, Sydney, Tokyo*

*Library of Congress Cataloging in Publication Data*

Novick, Barbara

Fundamentals of Clinical Child Neuropsychology / Barbara Novick

Maureen M. Arnold
p. cm.
Bibliography: p.
Includes index.ISBN 0-8089-1910-5
1. Pediatric neuropsychology. I. Arnold, Maureen M. II. Title.
[DNLM: 1. Child Development Disorders. 2. Nervous System Diseases—in infancy & childhood. 3. Neuropsychology—in infancy & childhood. WS 340 N943h]

RJ486.5.N68 1988 616.92'8—dc19

DNLM/DLC
for library of Congress 87-31487
CIP



Grune & Stratton

Philadelphia, PA 19106

Library of Congress Catalog Number 87-31487

International Standard Book Number 0-8089-1910-5

Printed in the United States of America
88 89 90 10 9 8 7 6 5 4 3 2 1

# ACKNOWLEDGMENTS

This book is a reflection of the influence of many individuals. Though it is not possible to mention all of them, several people deserve special thanks.

Lawrence Benjamin first introduced us to the theory and practice of clinical child neuropsychology and has been a valued colleague and friend for many years.

Our students and colleagues have provided an invaluable source of stimulation and encouragement. Their desire to learn more about this area has been crucial both in our decision to write this book and in our formulation of its organization and purpose.

We are indebted to our patients who have provided the rich clinical experience that is so vital to the bridging of theory and practice in clinical child neuropsychology

We are deeply grateful to our families for their firm support throughout this endeavor. Their support was very important to our own enthusiasm for this project. We also thank our colleagues at Lenox Hill Hospital and Albert Einstein College of Medicine for their interest and encouragement.

Several people read the manuscript and provided invaluable suggestions. Special thanks go to Richard Novick whose editorial expertise was so generously offered over many hours.

We are grateful for the guidance of Barbara Murphy, the Grune and Stratton editor responsible for Fundamentals of Clinical Child Neuropsychology.

B.Z.N.

M.M.A.

# CONTENTS

1

INTRODUCTION . . . . . 1

2

THE HUMAN NERVOUS SYSTEM . . . . . 3

3

TOPICS FOR SPECIAL CONSIDERATION: Brain Dysfunction, Critical Periods, Plasticity, Generalizations from Adults to Children, Handedness, and Mental Retardation . . . . . 26

4

LANGUAGE AND SPEECH DISORDERS . . . . . 34

5

EPISODIC DISORDERS: Epileptic Seizure Disorders, Seizure Disorders of Infancy and Childhood, and Headaches . . . . . 51

6

MEMORY DISORDERS . . . . . 66

7

SENSORY AND PERCEPTUAL DISORDERS . . . . . 76

8

MOTOR DISORDERS . . . . . 99

9

READING DISORDERS ........................................ 112

10

WRITING DISORDERS ........................................ 122

11

ARITHMETIC DISORDERS ........................................ 131

12

EMOTIONAL AND BEHAVIORAL DISORDERS ........................ 139

13

COMPREHENSIVE PSYCHOLOGICAL EVALUATION .................. 153

GLOSSARY ........................................ 159

APPENDICES

1. Distributors and Publishers of Tests ........................ 167
2. History ........................................ 168
3. School Report ........................................ 170
4. Clinical Observation ........................................ 173
5. Representative Quantitative and Qualitative Measures of Language Competence, Language Subskills and Speech ........................ 176
6. Representative Quantitative and Qualitative Measures of Memory ..... 177
7. Representative Quantitative and Qualitative Measures of Visual Disorders ........................................ 178
8. Representative Quantitative and Qualitative Measures of Auditory Disorders ........................................ 180
9. Representative Quantitative and Qualitative Measures of Touch and Body Schema Disorders ........................ 181
10. Representative Quantitative and Qualitative Measures of Motor Disorders ........................................ 183
11. Representative Quantitative and Qualitative Measures of Reading Competence ........................................ 185

12. Representative Quantitative and Qualitative Measures of Reading Subskills ... 187
13. Representative Quantitative and Qualitative Measures of Writing Competence ... 191
14. Representative Quantitative and Qualitative Measures of Writing Subskills ... 192
15. Representative Quantitative and Qualitative Measures of Arithmetic Competence ... 196
16. Representative Quantitative and Qualitative Measures of Arithmetic Subskills ... 197

SUGGESTED READINGS ... 202

INDEX ... 205

# 1

# INTRODUCTION

This book deals with the neuropsychological disorders of children (and adolescents). A neuropsychological disorder is typically defined as a disturbance in mental development or performance that is a consequence of a specific brain dysfunction. In contrast with global impairment of function, referred to as mental retardation, neuropsychological disorders are frequently subtle, and their delineation requires careful and insightful investigation in the problem area.

It has been estimated that more than five in every hundred children have a neuropsychological disorder of sufficient severity to interfere with cognitive development, school performance, and emotional well-being. The majority of these disorders are amenable to effective treatment if diagnosed early and treated optimally. Unfortunately, although the tools are now available to identify them, most neuropsychological disorders in children are poorly diagnosed. Without an accurate diagnosis, effective treatment is rare.

It is our view that an appreciation of the nature and evaluation of neuropsychological disorders is an important aspect of the mental health endeavor and should be included in undergraduate, graduate, and preprofessional curricula. Educators and health professionals who care for children should also be knowledgeable about these disorders.

This book is an attempt to outline the fundamental principles of clinical child neuropsychology in a simple and straightforward style. We have combined a concise presentation of complex biological systems with current understanding of brain-behavior relationships in a range of childhood disorders. Two general groups of disorders are discussed: those that are commonly seen in children and those that, though rarely seen, have heuristic value in the study of clinical child neuropsychology. The literature on adult neuropsychology is discussed in order to present both a historical perspective on the field and a crucial body of knowledge.

In order to provide sufficient depth in our overview of clinical child neuro-

FUNDAMENTALS OF CLINICAL CHILD NEUROPSYCHOLOGY

ISBN 0-8089-1910-5

psychology, which is a rich and rapidly expanding specialty area, we have had to limit the number of topics presented. Thus, we do not discuss closed head injury, neuropsychological assessment of preschool children, or the specific prescriptive treatment of individual problems. The omissions do not imply that given topics are either theoretically or practically unimportant. Rather, they reflect the authors' view that additional topics should be presented after the contents of an introductory guide such as ours have been fully appreciated.

Our book integrates the theoretical knowledge and clinical experience of the authors. Its content mirrors that of our courses and seminars, developed over many years of training students and colleagues in the neuropsychological evaluation of children as part of a comprehensive psychological evaluation.

The book is organized in the following manner. After an overview of the human nervous system, several topics are summarized for special consideration. These include brain dysfunction, critical periods, plasticity, difficulties in generalizing from adults to children, handedness, and mental retardation. We then discuss language and speech disorders, episodic disorders (seizures and headaches), memory disorders, sensory/perceptual, and motor disorders. Developmental reading disorders, writing disorders, and arithmetic disorders are presented next, followed by emotional and behavioral disorders. In the final chapter we expand on the nature of a comprehensive psychological evaluation and summarize the typical recommendations made by a psychologist on the basis of the evaluation findings. Individual chapters of the book are written to stand independently. A glossary is provided. Appendices list companies through which test materials can be purchased, and others outline actual clinical procedures referred to in the body of the text. Further readings are suggested at the end of the book.

In our own work, we assume an investigative approach to the diagnostic process. In such an approach, the diagnostician goes beyond a single test, test battery, or profile analysis in order to hone in on the specific brain-behavior disturbance in a child. Above all else, we hope that our readers come away from this book sharing our sense of the excitement and the power of an investigative approach. We also hope that they soon find themselves using such an approach in questioning old assumptions and developing new insights into the underlying causes of aberrant behavior in children.

The purpose of this book is three-fold. First, it is a guide for professionals who work with children (and adolescents) as diagnosticians, as therapists, and as teachers. Second, it is a comprehensive and concise aid to preparation for the neuropsychology component of the psychology licensing examination and the neuropsychology board examinations. Finally, it is an introductory textbook in clinical child neuropsychology for students at the undergraduate and graduate levels.

# 2

# THE HUMAN NERVOUS SYSTEM

In order to design, administer, and interpret a psychological diagnostic battery, the psychologist must possess basic knowledge of the human nervous system. In this chapter, we present an overview of the structural and functional organization of the human nervous system, discuss its component parts, and summarize a number of general principles of cerebral organization.

## ORGANIZATION

The human nervous system is made up of: (1) the cerebrum, (2) the deep cerebral structures, (3) the brain stem, (4) the cerebellum, (5) the spinal cord, and (6) the peripheral nerves. The cerebrum, deep cerebral structures, brain stem, and cerebellum make up the brain. A side view of the brain and spinal cord is diagrammed in Figure 2-1.

Structurally, the nervous system can be divided into two parts: (1) the central nervous system (CNS) and (2) the peripheral nervous system (PNS). The CNS is made up of the brain and the spinal cord. The PNS consists of the nerves that branch out from the brain (cranial nerves) and spinal cord, and portions of the autonomic nervous system, defined below.

The nervous system has two functional divisions: (1) the somatic and (2) the autonomic. The somatic system is made up of the structures that convey information to the CNS from the body (afferent) and from the CNS to the voluntary muscles (efferent). The somatic nervous system is comprised of the sensory receptors, the sensory pathways, the brain and spinal cord, motor pathways, and the neuromuscular endings

FUNDAMENTALS OF CLINICAL CHILD NEUROPSYCHOLOGY

ISBN 0-8089-1910-5

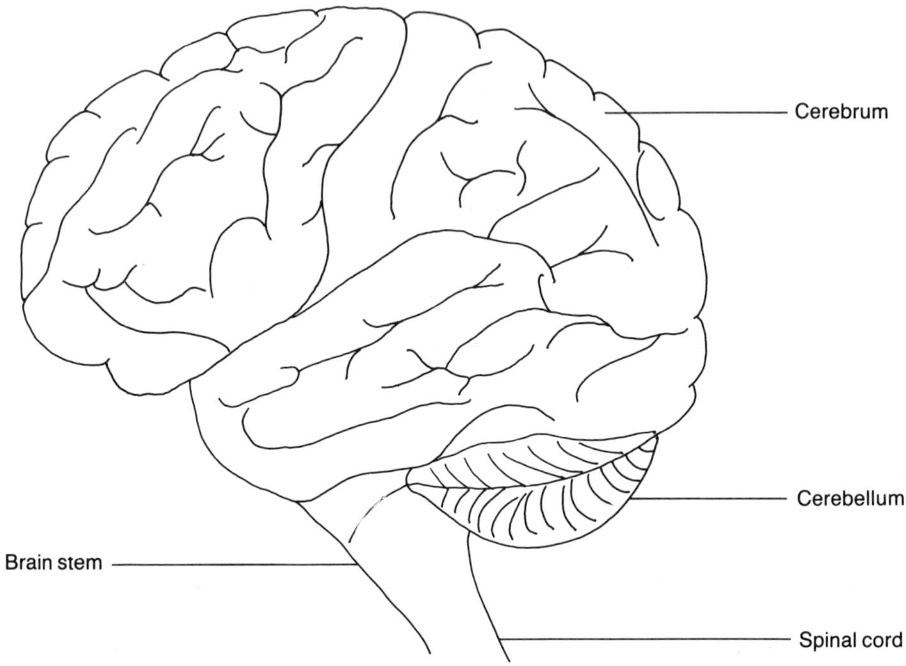


**Figure 2–1.** Side view of the brain and spinal cord.

of voluntary muscles in the head and body. The autonomic nervous system is responsible for conveying and processing information from the visceral organs and for motor control of the involuntary muscles, the muscles of the heart, and the secretory glands. It has stimulatory and inhibitory components known as sympathetic and parasympathetic systems, respectively.

This chapter focuses on the CNS and the somatic nervous system.

## THE NEURON

The neuron is the building block of the human nervous system. A neuron has three subdivisions: (1) the dendrite, (2) the cell body (soma), and (3) the axon. A schematic representation of a typical neuron is presented in Figure 2-2. The dendrite and axon are called nerve fibers, or nerve processes. Dendrites receive impulses from sensory receptors or other neurons; axons transmit nerve impulses to other nerve cells or to effector organs, such as skeletal muscles. The impulses are transmitted from one neuron to the next via neuronal junctions called synapses. A nerve is a collection of nerve fibers. Nerve fibers in the CNS are typically short and highly branched; PNS nerve

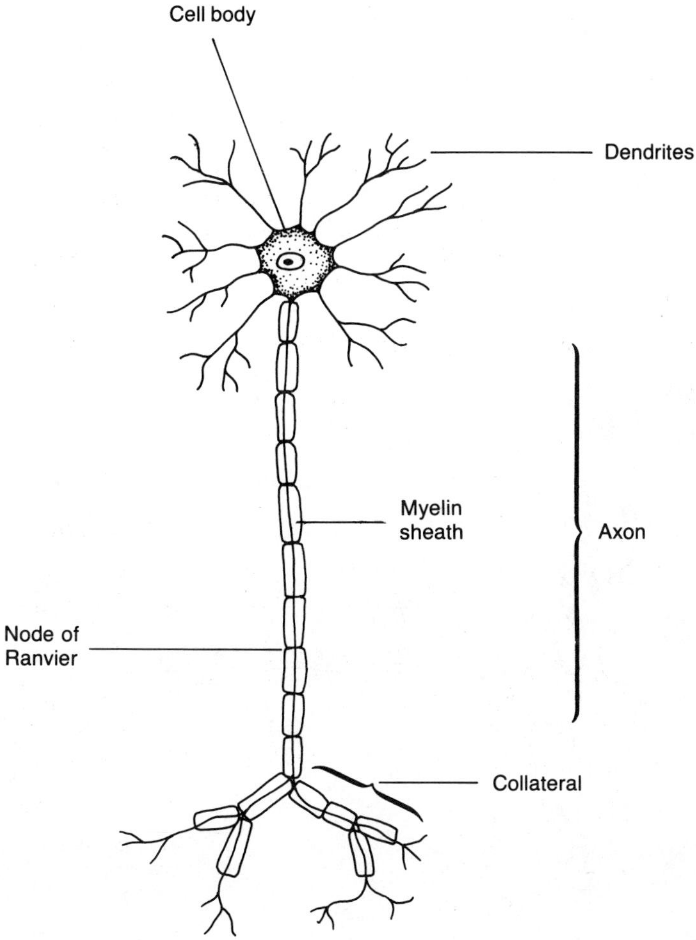


**Figure 2–2.** A typical neuron. (Reproduced from *Psychology* by H. Gleitman by permission of W. W. Norton & Company, Inc. Copyright © 1981 by W. W. Norton & Company, Inc.)

fibers are several feet long and are typically unbranched or may branch into a small number of collaterals.

Many nerve fibers are individually encased in sheaths of a fatty material known as myelin. Myelin insulates the fibers electrically. The myelin sheath is interrupted at regular intervals, called nodes of Ranvier. The nodes serve as relay stations. The rate of impulse transmission is increased by the impulse jumping from node to node. Fibers with thick myelin sheaths transmit more rapidly than those with thin sheaths. Myelination begins to appear between the fourth month of fetal life and the end of the first year of postnatal life. It starts in the spinal cord, then spreads.

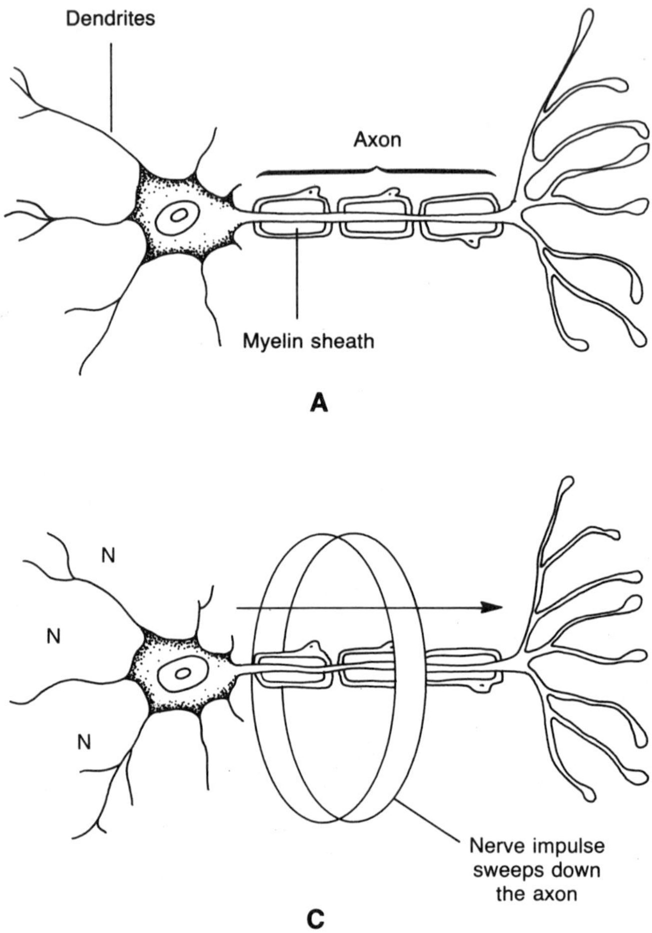


**Figure 2–3.** Interneuronal communication. (From *Understanding Human Behavior,* 5/e, by J. V. McConnell. Copyright © 1986 by CBS College Publishing. Reprinted by permission of Holt, Rinehart, & Winston, Inc.)

## Growth and Development of Neurons

Cell multiplication and cell differentiation characterize neuronal development during early fetal life. Differentiation of neuronal tissue consists of concurrent processes that include: (1) development of the cell body, (2) selective cell death, (3) development of the axons and dendrites, and (4) development of synapses.

The majority of neurons are fully developed by early postnatal life. During the life span, they are not replaced. An exception is the neurons of the olfactory nerve, which are continually dying and being replaced.

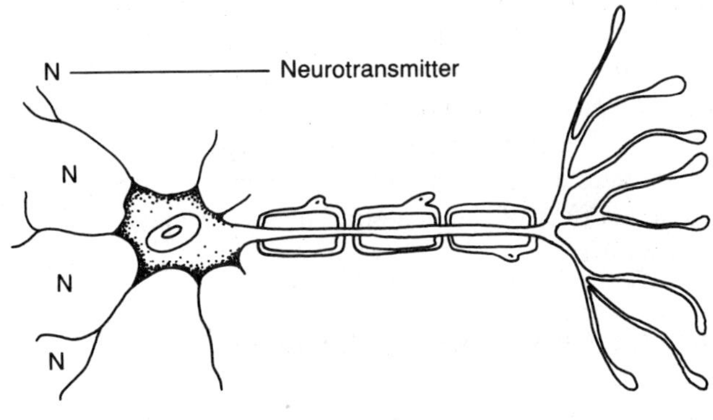


B

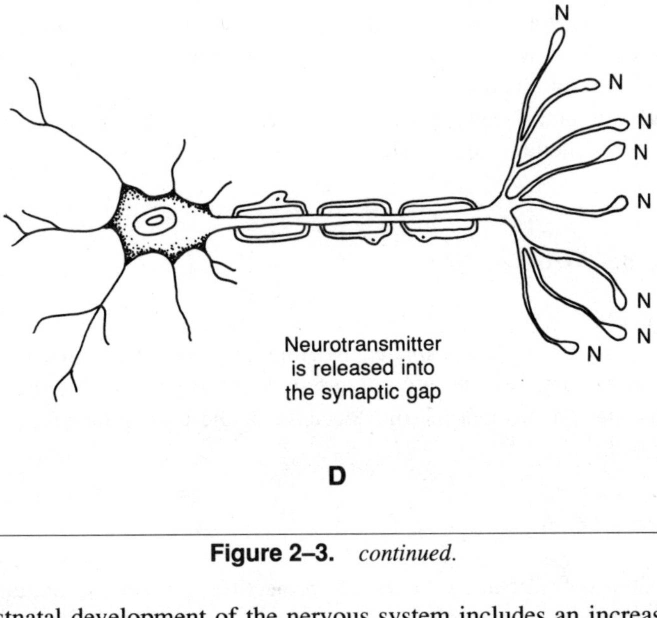


D

**Figure 2–3.** *continued.*

Later postnatal development of the nervous system includes an increase in: (1) the size of the neurons, (2) the number of interneuronal connections, and (3) myelination.

## Interneuronal Communication

The fundamental unit of the nervous system is the neuronal circuit, through which information traverses a chain of neurons in the form of a nerve impulse. A nerve impulse is an electrochemical process that originates in the cell body, triggered by stimuli that are above a threshold value. The impulse travels out along the axon.

Interneuronal communication takes place at the synapse. Presynaptic membranes of transmitting neurons are located at the ends of axons. Postsynaptic membranes of receiving neurons are located on dendrites and on cell bodies. Synaptic transmission occurs through the release of a chemical (a neurotransmitter) at the presynaptic membrane (see Figure 2-3). Neurotransmitters include acetylcholine, dopamine, epinephrine, and norepinephrine. The neurotransmitter crosses the gap between neurons (synaptic cleft) and is picked up by receptor sites on the postsynaptic membrane. Receptor sites are spots on the dendrites or cell body that are sensitive to neurotransmitters. The effect of the neurotransmitter on the next nerve cell may be either excitatory or inhibitory.

## Types of Cells in the Central Nervous System

There are two major structural classes of neurons in the CNS, known as Golgi type I and Golgi type II. Golgi type I cells are usually large, with long axons and multiple branched dendrites. They are thought to form prenatally and to represent the majority of neurons in the nervous system. Golgi type II cells, in contrast, are usually small, with small axons and dendrites. They are thought to form postnatally and to be important for higher cerebral functions.

The CNS also contains cells that are not neurons. Called neuroglia, or glial cells, these cells serve structural and nutritional roles in the system. They also form the myelin sheaths.

## Gray Matter and White Matter

One way in which regions of the nervous system are identified is by the preponderance of gray matter or white matter. Regions that consist of closely packed unmyelinated nerve fibers, grayish in color, are called gray matter. Regions that consist of nerve fibers that are whitish in color because of the preponderance of myelin are called white matter.

## Types of Nerve Fibers

There are three types of nerve fibers: (1) projection, (2) association, and (3) commissural.

Nerve fibers that connect different areas of the CNS are called projection fibers. They are divided into two functional classes: (1) afferent and (2) efferent. The afferent nerve fibers transmit information toward or into the CNS. They are attached to or are extensions of receptor cells which respond to various stimuli, such as pressure, light, and sound. They are also known as sensory nerve fibers. The efferent, or motor, nerve fibers carry information out of the CNS to effector organs. Nearly all nerves contain both afferent and efferent nerve fibers.

Association fibers connect neurons within the brain, and they also connect neurons within the spinal cord. They are typically characterized by considerable branching of both the dendrites and the axons, having a large number of synapses. Association neurons, also called interneurons, are the most numerous type of neuron in the CNS. They connect two neurons in a circuit.

Opposite areas of the two cerebral hemispheres are connected by commissural fibers, discussed below.

## THE CENTRAL NERVOUS SYSTEM

During embryonic development, what is to become the CNS evolves as a tubular structure, the neural tube. The part of the tube in the head region becomes the brain. The rest of the tube becomes the spinal cord.

### The Brain

The neural tube in the head region forms three enlargements: (1) the forebrain, (2) the midbrain, and (3) the hindbrain. In the course of development, the forebrain forms the endbrain (telencephalon) and the interbrain (diencephalon). The telencephalon evolves to become the cerebrum. The midbrain (mescencephalon) remains the midbrain. The hindbrain forms the pons, medulla, and cerebellum.

The brain is protected by layers of skin, bone, membrane (meninges), and fluid (cerebrospinal fluid). It is fed oxygen and glucose via blood delivered by the circulatory system.

#### *Forebrain*

**CEREBRUM.** The cerebrum comprises two cerebral hemispheres, which are divided into regions on the basis of structural and functional criteria.

***Structural.*** The cerebral hemispheres are subdivided on the basis of physical demarcations apparent on the surface, or cortex. The cortex is deeply folded and convoluted. Sulci (valleys) and gyri (ridges) on the surface are used as landmarks.

Along the center of the cerebral cortex lies the longitudinal sulcus, which divides the cortex into two hemispheres. On each cerebral hemisphere, lesser "valleys" are found. One of these, the central sulcus, runs laterally and downward from the top of the hemisphere. Another, the Sylvian fissure, runs along the lower region of the cortex, at one point meeting the central sulcus. Physical demarcations divide the cortex into four regions, or lobes: (1) the occipital lobe, (2) the temporal lobe, (3) the parietal lobe, and (4) the frontal lobe. The occipital and parietal lobes lie behind the central sulcus. The temporal lobe is below the Sylvian fissure. The frontal lobe is in front of the central sulcus.

Gyri are often used to delineate regions within the lobes; for example, the angular gyrus is located at the juncture of the temporal and parietal lobes, adjacent to the occipital lobe. A diagram of the surface of the cerebral cortex, showing the major demarcations, is presented in Figure 2-4.

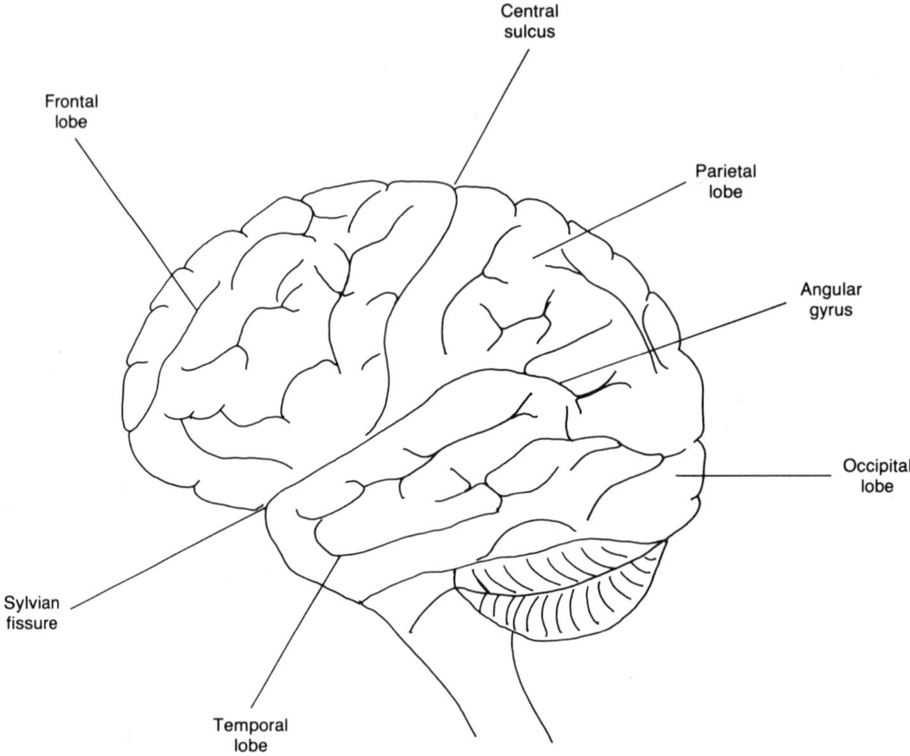


**Figure 2–4.** The cerebral cortex, showing major demarcations and lobes.

***Functional Regions.*** The central sulcus divides the cerebral cortex into posterior and anterior regions. The posterior region comprises the occipital, temporal, and parietal lobes; the anterior region, the frontal lobe. Functionally, the posterior portion is the sensory area of the cerebral cortex; the anterior region is the motor area and the area responsible for planned behavior. Brodmann's system, used to reference cortical areas in the discussion below, is presented in Figure 2-5.

*Posterior Cerebral Cortex.* The posterior cerebral cortex is divided functionally into projection and association areas. Sensory information from the internal and external environments is received and processed in this region. The projection zone mediates the intitial reception of incoming information. The association region has discriminative and integrative functions, imposing meaning on the information based on past experiences and learning. There is functional asymmetry between the two cerebral hemispheres at the association level.

**Figure 2–5.** Cortical areas referenced by Brodmann's system. *A*, Lateral surface. *B*, Medial surface. (Adapted with permission from *The Nervous System*, 3/e, by C. R. Noback and R. J. Demarest. McGraw-Hill Book Company, 1986.)

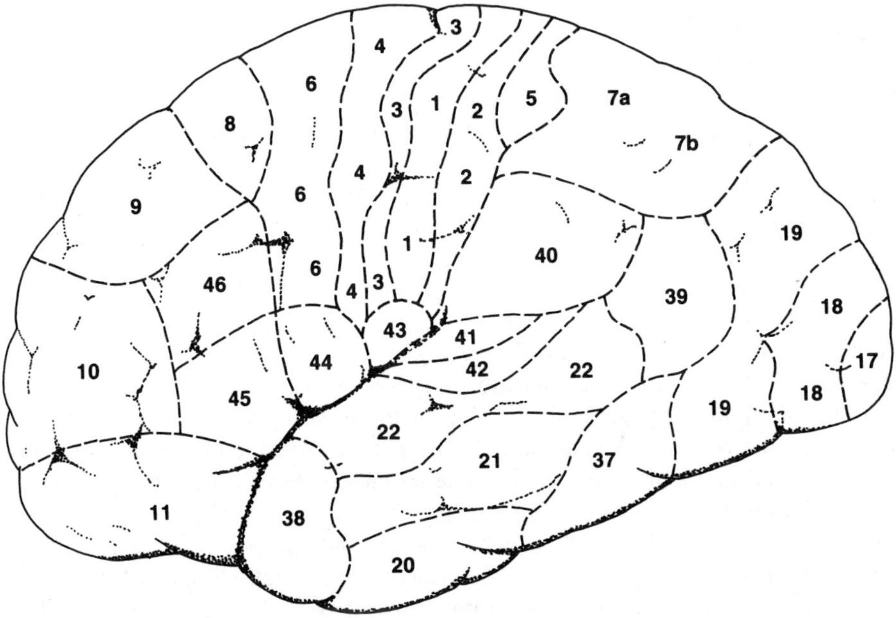


A Lateral surface

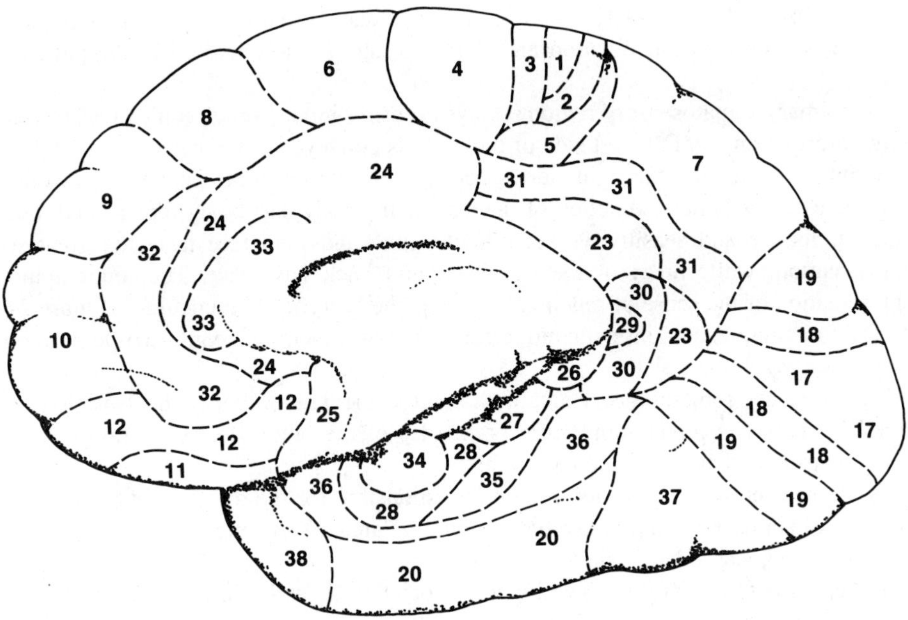


B Medial surface

Higher level association zones lie in the areas of overlap between the lobes. They are not modality specific in function. Rather, they mediate the integration of information across the modalities.

*Sensory Areas.* The three sensory areas are: (1) visual, (2) auditory, and (3) somatosensory. The visual cortex includes the primary visual zone (area 17) and the visual association area (areas 18 and 19), located in the occipital lobe. Within the primary visual cortex, input from both eyes is fused into one image, and the orientation of visual stimuli in the visual field is appreciated. The visual association area is responsible for interpreting visual images. Damage to this area results in impaired interpretation of visual stimuli.

The auditory cortex includes the primary auditory zone (area 41) and the auditory association region (areas 22 and 42). These areas are located in the temporal lobe. The primary auditory cortex is tonotopically organized, i.e., responses to different frequencies (high vs. low) are in different locations. Although transmission of auditory information to the brain is primarily to the side of the brain opposite the receiving ear (contralateral representation), some information is transmitted to the same side of the brain (ipsilateral representation). Thus, bilateral damage results in cortical deafness; unilateral damage results in a rise in hearing threshold.

The auditory association region mediates the interpretation of sounds. The language-dominant hemisphere (usually the left) discriminates auditory stimuli as they relate to language; the right hemisphere processes nonverbal acoustical stimuli. Impaired language functions are the consequence of dysfunction in this region of the language-dominant cerebral hemisphere. Right hemispheric dysfunction results in impaired ability to perceive complex nonverbal acoustic stimuli.

The somatosensory cortex (also referred to as the sensory cortex) includes the primary sensory zone (areas 1, 2, and 3), the secondary somatosensory area (area 43), and the somatosensory association area (areas 5 and 7). It is located in the parietal lobe.

The primary somatosensory region receives sensory input from specific areas of the body. Information from the left side of the body is conveyed to the right parietal lobe, while information from the right side is conveyed to the left lobe. Spatial representation in the cortex is not a function of the size of the body part being represented, but rather of its use and sensitivity. Accordingly, the hands and face have the greatest representation, while areas of the shoulders and back have less. The topographic representation of the sense of touch is known as the "sensory homunculus" (Figure 2-6). Dysfunction results in deficited discriminative functions (e.g., two-point discrimination).

The secondary somatosensory area is thought to mediate primarily the sensation of pain. This region receives input from both sides of the body. Representation in this region is ipsilateral as well as contralateral.

The somatosensory association region is responsible for the discrimination and integration of somesthetic input. Dysfunction in this area affects interpretation of tactile stimulation (e.g., agraphesthesia).

*Higher Association Areas.* The higher association areas lie in the juncture of the

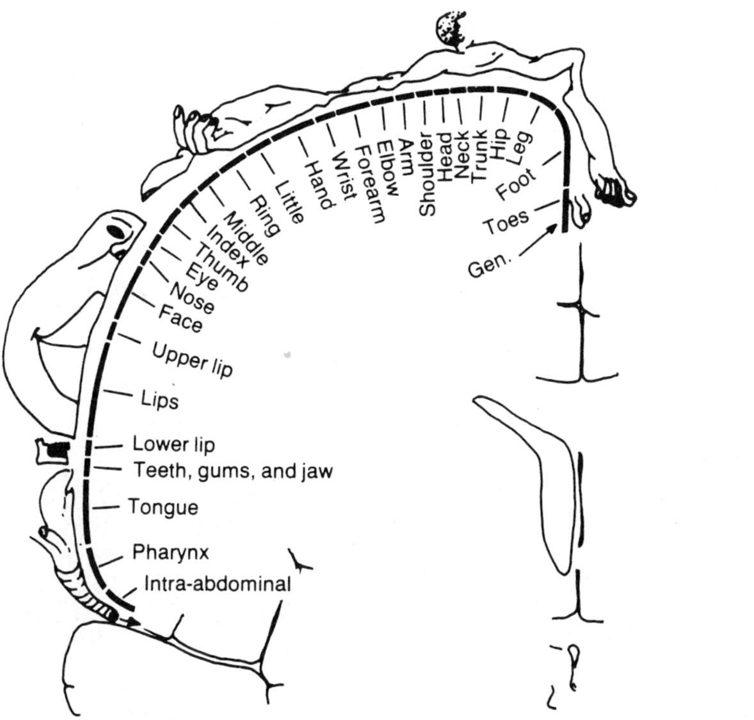


**Figure 2–6.** Sensory homunculus. (Reprinted with permission of Macmillan Publishing Company from *The Cerebral Cortex of Man* by W. Penfield and T. Rasmussen. Copyright © 1950 by Macmillan Publishing Company, renewed 1978 by Theodore Rasmussen.)

temporal and occipital lobes (area 37), the temporal lobe (areas 21 and 22), and the parietal lobe (areas 7, 39, and 40). These regions perform the highest level of integration of information from all the senses. Dysfunction in the language-dominant hemisphere is manifested by deficited complex language based functions. Dysfunction in the right hemisphere results in deficient integration of visual-spatial and nonlinguistic material.

*Anterior Cerebral Cortex.* The anterior cerebral cortex mediates the formulation, execution, evaluation, and modification of behavior (motor and nonmotor). The region is organized hierarchically into projection areas and higher association regions.

*Motor Areas.* The motor cortex includes the primary motor zone (area 4), the **premotor cortex** (areas 6 and 8), and the supplementary motor area (area 44). These are located in the frontal lobe.

The primary motor zone, located in the precentral gyrus of the frontal lobe, has the most direct link to the effector organs, i.e., the muscles. The face and body are represented contralaterally and in proportion to the fineness of motor control required of the body part. The "motor homunculus" depicts the representational pattern (Figure 2-7).

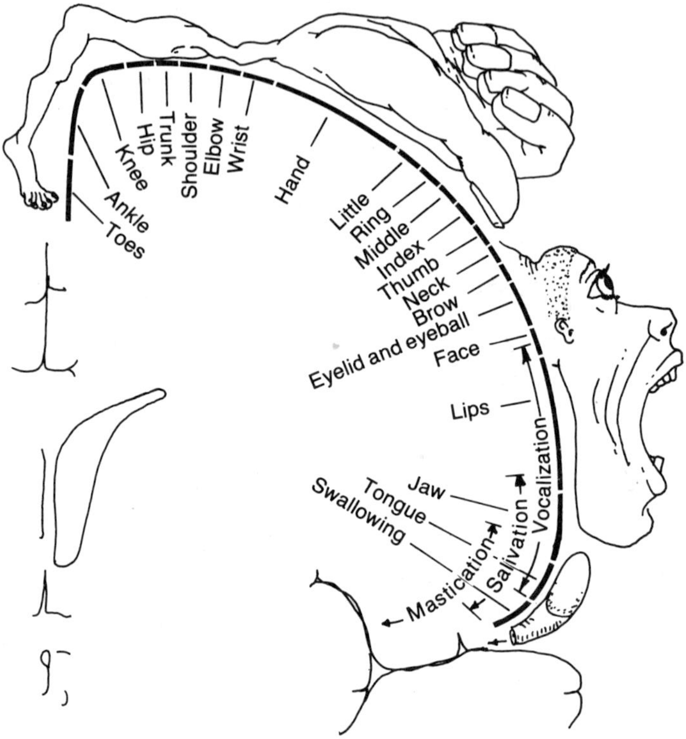


**Figure 2–7.** Motor homunculus. (Reprinted with permission of Macmillan Publishing Company from *The Cerebral Cortex of Man* by W. Penfield and T. Rasmussen. Copyright © 1950 by Macmillan Publishing Company, renewed 1978 by Theodore Rasmussen.)

The premotor cortex integrates individual movements into larger functional units. The area is divided into two regions, one mediating movement of most of the body (area 6), the second (area 8), movement of the head and eyes. The supplementary motor area (area 44) is associated with movement of the oral musculature.

*Higher Association Area.* The higher association area is located in the prefrontal cortex. This region is divided into the dorsolateral area (areas 9, 10, 11, 45, and 46) and the orbital area (areas 11, 12, 34, and 47). The prefrontal cortex is responsible for: (1) the highest level of integration of information from the external and internal environments, (2) the planning and organization of sequential behavior, and (3) the evaluation and modification of behavior. Dysfunction in this region results in disorders involving regulation of affect, cognition and planned behavior.

## DEEP CEREBRAL STRUCTURES

***Diencephalon.*** The diencephalon region lies within the cerebral hemispheres. It includes: (1) the thalamus and (2) the hypothalamus. The functions of the thalamus include acting as a relay station for all the sensory information (except smell) transmit-

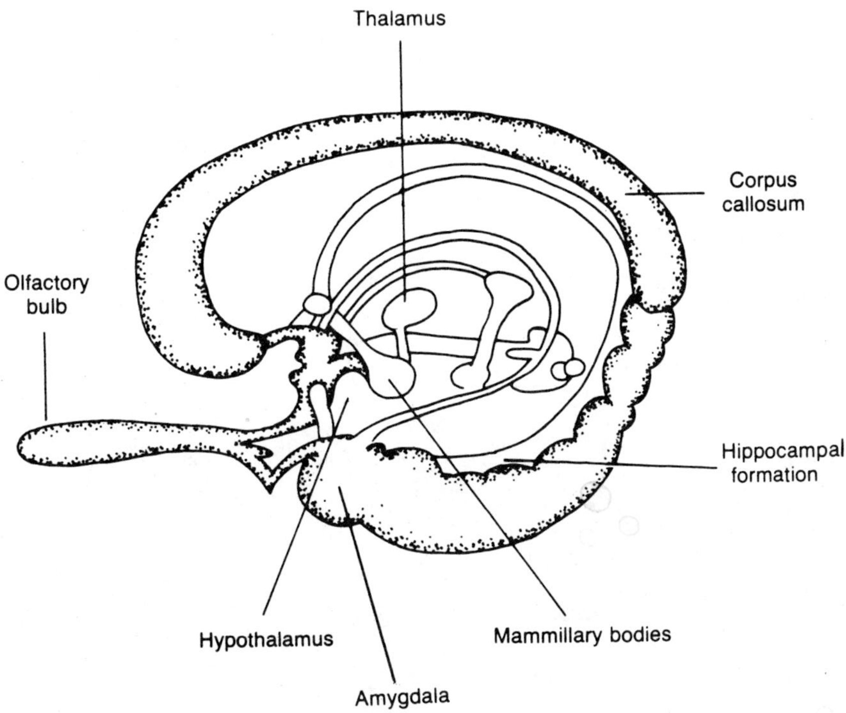


**Figure 2–8.** Major structures of the limbic system. (Adapted with permission from *Clinical Neuropsychology*, 2/e, by K. Heilman and E. Valenstein. Oxford University Press, 1985.)

ted to the cerebral cortex. The hypothalamus has regulating functions, such as influencing appetite, sexual arousal, and emotional behavior. Part of the thalamus and the hypothalamus are part of the limbic system, discussed below. Located also within the diencephalon are the pituitary gland, the pineal gland, and mammillary bodies.

***The Basal Ganglia.*** The basal ganglia, or basal nuclei, are masses of gray matter in the interior of the cerebrum, lying predominantly above the diencephalon.

The basal ganglia function as a processing station, or bridge, between the sensory and motor systems. In combination with other structures of the brain, they influence motor activity.

***Limbic System.*** The limbic system is made up of the limbic lobe and areas of cortical and subcortical gray matter. The limbic system includes the hippocampal formation, olfactory bulb, mammillary bodies, the amygdala, part of the thalamus, and the hypothalamus. The structures of the limbic system are organized in complex loops or circuits.

The limbic system mediates behavior that is basic to the survival of the individual and the preservation of the species, such as emotions, memory, feeding behavior, and reproductive behavior. Major structures of the limbic system are diagrammed in Figure 2-8.

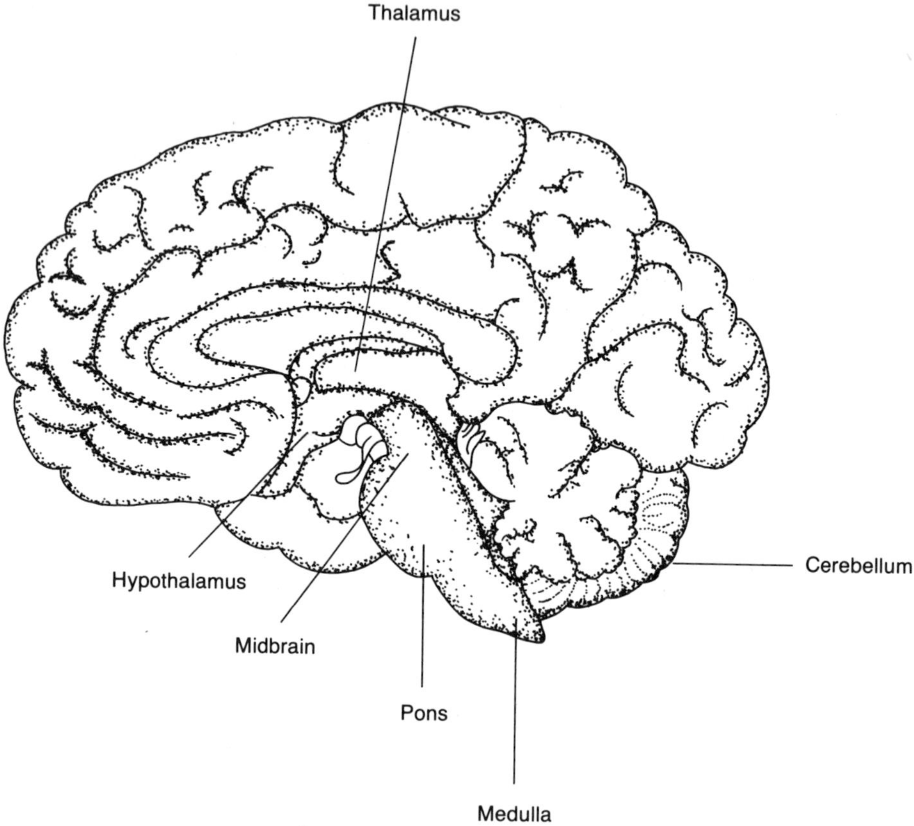


**Figure 2–9.** Inner structures of the brain, brain stem, and cerebellum. (Adapted with permission from *Dyslexia: Neuropsychological Theory, Research, and Clinical Differentiation* by G. Hynd and M. Cohen. Grune & Stratton, Inc., 1983.)

### *Midbrain and Hindbrain*

The midbrain, or mescencephalon, is a relatively small stalk connecting the forebrain and the hindbrain. The principal parts of the hindbrain are the medulla, the pons, and the cerebellum. The brain stem comprises the midbrain, pons, and medulla.

**BRAIN STEM.** The brain stem lies between the inner core of the cerebrum and the spinal cord. The brain stem contains: (1) the long nerve tracts that carry sensory and motor impulses between the body and the brain; (2) the nuclei of the majority of the cranial nerves; and (3) the vital systems concerned with vigilance, sleep, motor tone, and autonomic functions. The reticular activating system (RAS) is one such system. The RAS receives and integrates information from a number of neural structures. The descending pathways mediate selective attention; the ascending pathways mediate cortical arousal.

**CEREBELLUM.** The cerebellum ("little brain") is a large structure lying at the base of the cerebrum, behind the brain stem. The cerebellum consists of two deeply convoluted hemispheres and a midline structure called the vermis. The cerebellum controls equilibrium (body balance) and muscle tone. The precision and coordination of motor activities are also mediated by the cerebellum. The influence of the cerebellum on balance and coordination is thought to be an inhibitory one. Motor disorders are ipsilateral to the site of the dysfunction.

Figure 2-9 depicts inner structures of the brain, the brain stem, and the cerebellum.

### The Spinal Cord

The spinal cord is a cylinder of white and gray matter. The white matter consists of the nerve fibers of the (descending) motor system and several (ascending) sensory systems—-those mediating position, vibration, pain, and touch. The gray matter contains: (1) the bodies of certain sensory and motor neurons and interneurons; (2) the synapses between peripheral sensory nerves and the neurons of the CNS; and (3) the synapses of the corticospinal tract and of the motor neurons within the spinal cord.

The spinal cord has two functions: (1) it serves as a pathway and a relay station for the afferent and efferent nerves coursing to and from the brain; and (2) it mediates the spinal reflexes.

Sensory information travels to the brain, and motor information travels from the brain through the spinal cord. Dysfunction at any level of the spinal cord will interrupt sensory impulses from the body innervated by nerves below the lesion and will block impulses from the brain to these same areas.

Spinal reflexes are divided into 3 groups: (1) deep tendon reflexes (DTR), (2) superficial reflexes, and (3) pathological reflexes.

Deep tendon reflexes or stretch reflexes are elicited by striking a tendon. An example of a deep tendon reflex is the knee jerk.

Superficial reflexes are elicited by stimulation of the skin. An example of a superficial reflex is the flexing of the toes when the soles of the feet are stroked.

Abnormal, or pathological, reflexes are responses that, unlike the DTR's and superficial reflexes, are not normally found in an individual over the age of one year. An example of a pathological reflex is the Babinski sign. The Babinski reflex is obtained by stroking along the side of the foot from the heel, crossing to the base of the great toe, with a sharp-edged object. The normal response is the flexion of all the toes (flexor response) or, in some cases, no response. The abnormal response— Babinski sign— is the dorsiflexion of the great toe and fanning of the other toes. The normal response and pathological sign are illustrated in Figure 2-10.

## THE PERIPHERAL NERVOUS SYSTEM

The peripheral nervous system (PNS) consists of: (1) cranial nerves, (2) spinal nerves, and (3) certain portions of the autonomic nervous system.

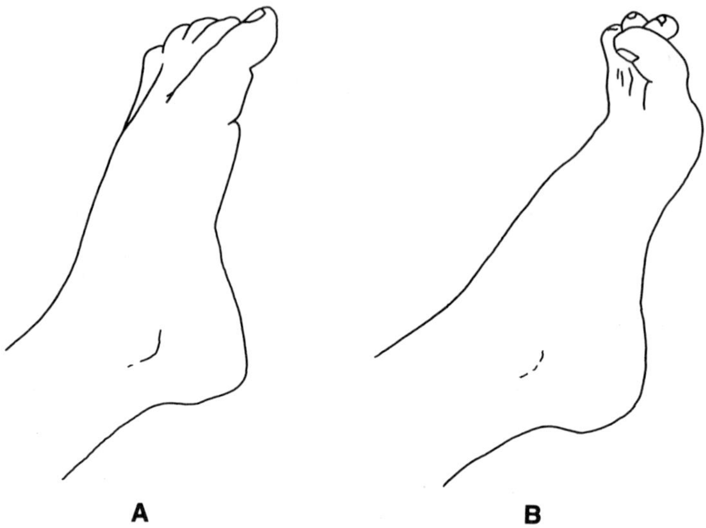


**Figure 2–10.** *A*. Normal response to the stimulation of the sole of the foot. *B*. Pathological response. (From *Fundamentals of Neurology* by E. Gardner. Copyright © 1964 by W. B. Saunders Co. Reprinted by permission of Holt, Rinehart, & Winston, Inc.)

## Cranial Nerves

Some cranial nerves carry afferent fibers; some carry efferent fibers; others carry both. The majority of the cranial nerves originate in the brain stem. Only the olfactory and optic nerves originate in the cerebrum.

Cranial nerves innervate the head, the neck region, and some visceral areas. The names and functions of the cranial nerves are presented in Table 2-1.

## Spinal Nerves

Spinal nerves transmit nerve impulses from the sense receptors and to the muscles and glands of the body. They arise from plexi formed by the nerves that radiate from the spinal cord. They are part of the somatic and autonomic nervous systems.

## Autonomic Nervous System

The autonomic nervous system functions automatically and reflexively, having a large degree of independence from the CNS. It sends commands to the glands and smooth muscles of the skin, the visceral organs (e.g., heart, stomach), and the blood vessels (Figure 2-11).

The autonomic nervous system has two divisions: (1) sympathetic and (2) parasympathetic. The sympathetic system activates the organism, placing it on emer-

**TABLE 2-1. THE CRANIAL NERVES AND THEIR FUNCTIONS**

| CRANIAL NERVE NO. | NAME | FUNCTION |
|---|---|---|
| I | Olfactory | Smell |
| II | Optic | Vision |
| III | Oculomotor | Eye movement; ocular reflexes |
| IV | Trochlear | Eye movement |
| V | Trigeminal | Facial senses; mastication |
| VI | Abducens | Eye movement |
| VII | Facial | Facial expression; lacrimation; salivation; taste |
| VIII | Acoustic -vestibular | Hearing; balance |
| IX | Glossopharyngeal | Swallowing; taste |
| X | Vagus | Reflexes and senses of the viscera; taste |
| XI | Accessory | Head and shoulder movement |
| XII | Hypoglossal | Tongue movement |

gency alert. It accelerates the heart and lung functions, triggers the conversion of foods in preparation for muscular efforts, and suppresses digestive and sexual activity. The parasympathetic system facilitates the vegetative functions of the body, i.e., the conservation of body resources, the elimination of wastes, and reproduction. The two systems never act independently but rather coordinate to maintain homeostasis (Table 2-2).

## GENERAL CONCEPTS OF CEREBRAL ORGANIZATION

### Cerebral Lateralization

Cerebral lateralization refers to asymmetry of function between the two cerebral hemispheres. Although structurally and functionally similar in many ways, the cerebral hemispheres have developed distinct areas of specialization. Lateralization of function is manifested in the left hemispheric specialization for: (1) language

**TABLE 2-2. FUNCTIONS OF THE SYMPATHETIC AND PARASYMPATHETIC DIVISIONS OF THE AUTONOMIC NERVOUS SYSTEM**

| ORGAN | SYMPATHETIC | PARASYMPATHETIC |
|---|---|---|
| *Eye* | Pupil dilatated | Pupil constricted |
| *Lacrimal, Nasal, Salivary Glands* | No important effect | Secretions stimulated |
| *Heart* | Heart rate increased | Heart rate slowed |
| *Lungs* | Mixed pattern | Breathing slowed |
| *Alimentary Canal* | Digestion inhibited | Digestion stimulated |
| *Adrenal Gland* | Secretion of epinephrine stimulated | No effect |
| *Colon and Bladder* | Evacuation inhibited | Evacuation stimulated |
| *Sweat glands* | Stimulated | No effect |
| *Smooth Muscles of Skin* | Erection of hairs and “goose bumps” stimulated | No effect |
| *Peripheral Blood Vessels* | Constricted and dilatated | No effect |

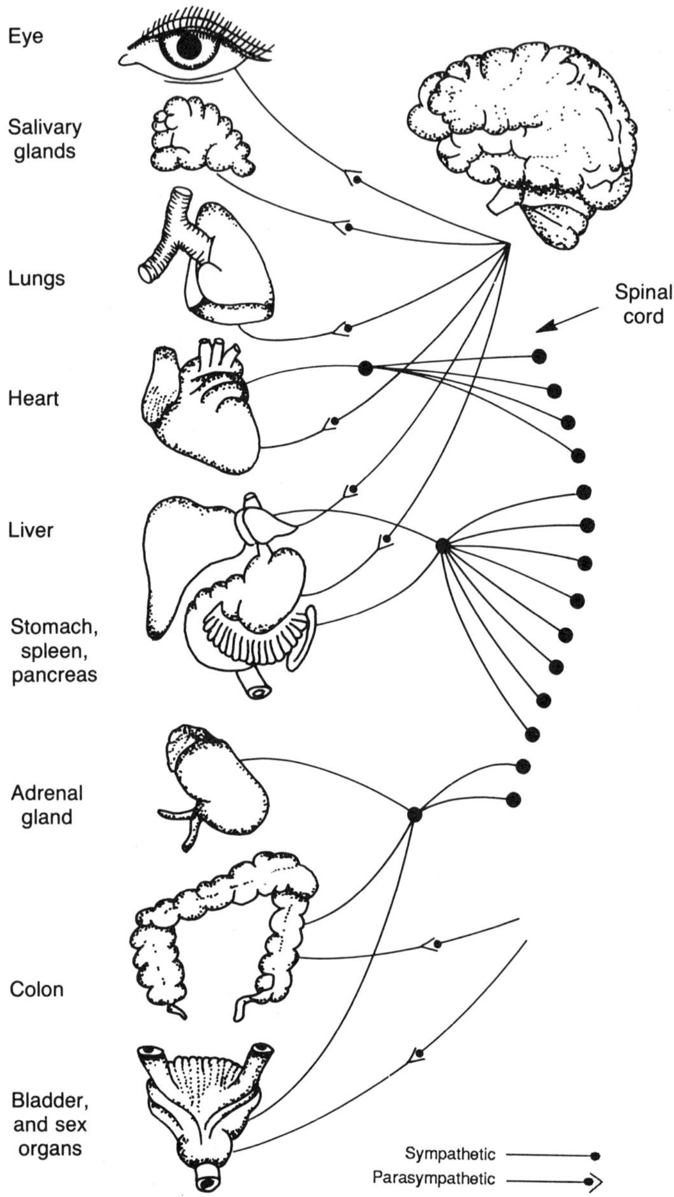


**Figure 2–11.** Organs of the autonomic nervous system. (From *Understanding Human Behavior*, 5/e, by J. V. McConnell. Copyright © 1986 by CBS College Publishing. Reprinted by permission of Holt, Rinehart, & Winston, Inc.)

functions in right-handers and the majority of left-handers and (2) the processing of serial information. The left hemisphere is often called the dominant hemisphere because of the lateralization of language functions in most individuals.

The right hemisphere of the cerebral cortex is specialized for: (1) visual perceptual tasks, including facial recognition; (2) nonverbal ideation; (3) the processing of nonspeech sounds, such as music; and (4) specific language functions, such as the rhythm of speech.

### *Evidence for Cerebral Lateralization*

Important evidence for cerebral lateralization of functions is derived from such sources as: (1) early clinicoanatomical studies of acquired language disorders, (2) split-brain research, and (3) dichotic listening studies.

Cerebral lateralization was first suggested by early work with adults who had acquired language disorders. Such studies gave rise to the hypothesis that the left hemisphere was responsible for language functions.

Further evidence for lateralization of functions came from studies of individuals with split brains. These are individuals who, due to intractable epilepsy, undergo split-brain surgery (commissurotomy), in which the corpus callosum, a bundle of fibers connecting the two hemispheres, is severed. As a consequence of this procedure, the two hemispheres are functionally isolated from each other.

The effect of the split-brain operation is demonstrated by posing a question to one side of the brain that requires the other side of the brain to respond. For example, when a normal individual is asked to label a visual stimulus, which is presented either to the right or left visual fields, he is able to respond. However, an individual with a commissurotomy can name a stimulus presented to the right visual field but not one presented to the left visual field. Without the commissures connecting the hemispheres, information arriving at the right occipital lobe cannot be transferred to the left hemisphere where it is labeled (Figure 2-12).

In the dichotic listening technique, competing messages are presented simultaneously to the two ears (see Figure 2-13). The presented messages may be verbal (e.g., words) or nonverbal (e.g., melodies). The individual is to report what he has heard. If the individual reports the information presented to one ear more accurately than that presented to the other, the cerebral hemisphere contralateral to the ear receiving the message is considered dominant for processing that type of information. Studies indicate that verbal messages are perceived more reliably when presented to the right ear. Nonverbal messages are perceived more accurately by the left ear.

### *Development of Cerebral Lateralization*

The development of lateralized cerebral function remains a controversial and widely debated topic. There are two major viewpoints. One holds that lateralization of higher cortical functions develops before birth. The degree of lateralization in the immature

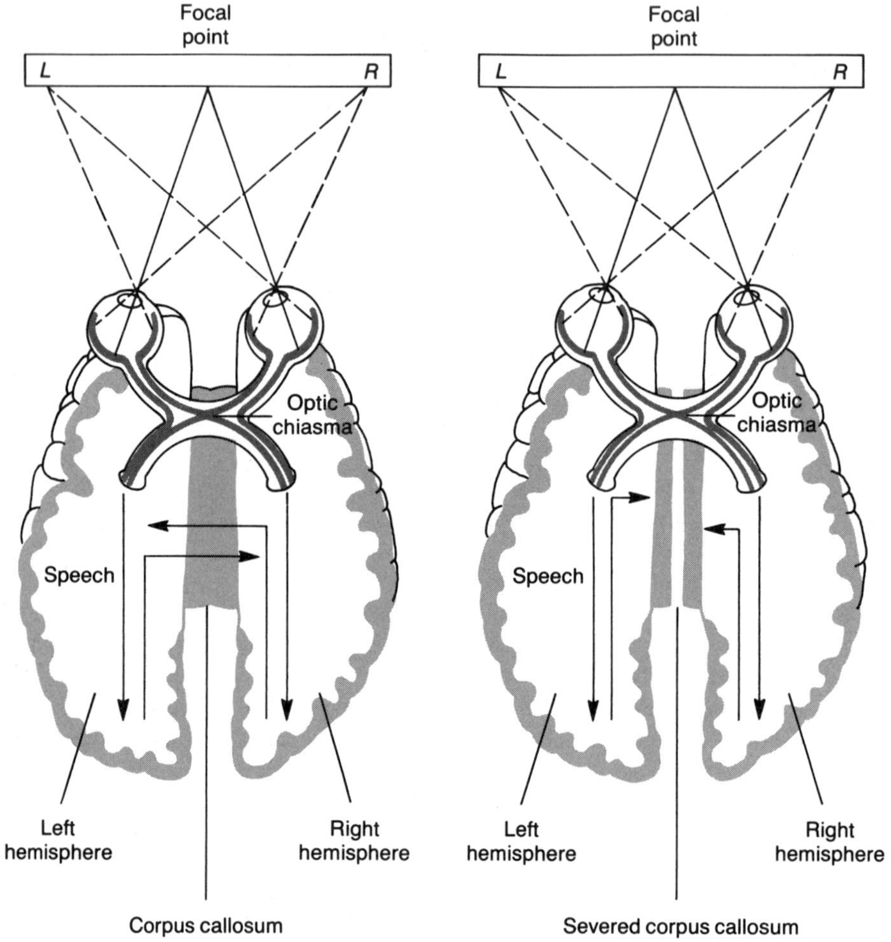


**Figure 2–12.** Neuroanatomical basis of the split-brain effect. (Reproduced from *Psychology* by H. Gleitman by permission of W. W. Norton & Company, Inc. Copyright © 1981 by W. W. Norton & Company, Inc.

brain and in the mature brain should, therefore, be the same. This view is commonly referred to as the invariant lateralization theory.

The second theory, in contrast, holds that most higher mental functions are controlled equally by both hemispheres at birth. As the brain matures, a majority of these functions shift to the left cerebral hemisphere. This results in the left hemisphere having a dominant role in later higher cortical activity. This view is referred to as the progressive lateralization theory.

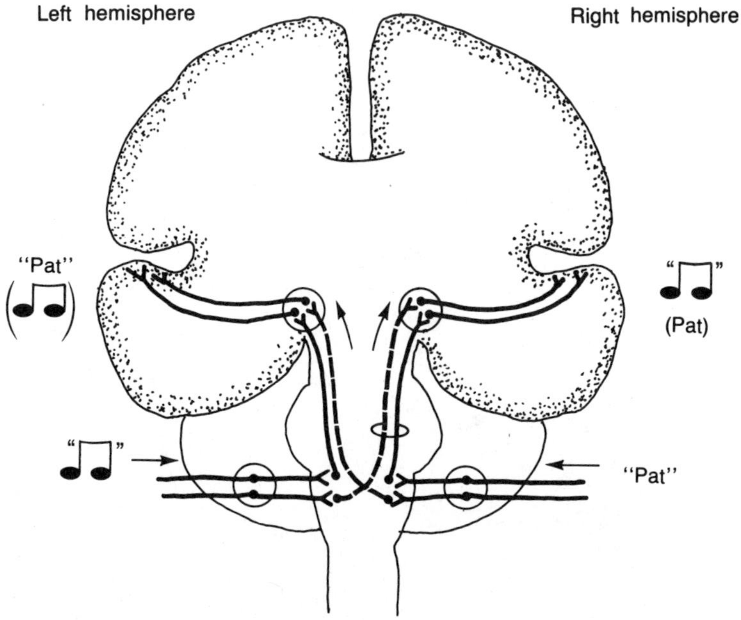


**Figure 2–13.** Auditory pathways involved in the dichotic listening effect. (Adapted from *Fundamentals of Neurology* by E. Gardner. Copyright © 1964 by W. B. Saunders Co. Reprinted by permission of Holt, Rinehart, & Winston, Inc.)

### *Interhemispheric Communication*

In order to perform complex tasks, then, the brain must integrate information from both hemispheres. For example, the task of copying a geometric design in pencil begins with visual analysis of the geometric shape. This is a right hemispheric function. If an individual is right-handed, motor control of his drawing hand is in the left hemisphere. Clearly, there must be communication between the cerebral hemispheres in order to perform such a task.

Information is transferred between the cerebral hemispheres via the interhemispheric commissures. Commissures are large fiber bundles that connect major regions of the cortex and are among the last brain structures to be myelinated.

The largest commissure is the corpus callosum, which connects the majority of the cortical regions of the two cerebral hemispheres. Another, smaller commissure, the anterior commissure, primarily connects anterior temporal lobes of the left and the right hemispheres (Figure 2-14).

In the split-brain surgical procedure (commissurotomy), the interhemispheric commissures are severed. As a result of the procedure, the two hemispheres function independently of one another. It is impossible to transfer information from one hemisphere to another, so that integrated functioning is precluded. The resulting behavioral

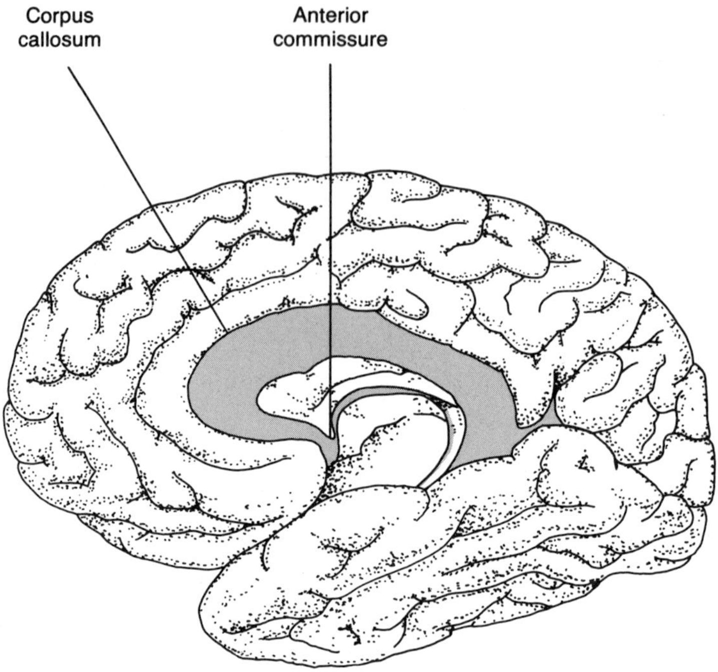


**Figure 2–14.** Commissures: corpus callosum and anterior commissure. (Reproduced from *Psychology* by H. Gleitman by permission of W. W. Norton & Company, Inc. Copyright © 1981 by W. W. Norton & Company, Inc.)

disturbance is known as the commissural disconnection syndrome. This syndrome can also be caused by a tumor or an interruption in the blood flow to the corpus callosum.

### *Ipsilateral and Contralateral Cortical Representation*

**AFFERENT PATHWAYS.** As a general rule, afferent pathways to the brain transmit information to the side opposite the point of stimulation. For example, the nerve impulse triggered by a light touch on the right arm is transmitted to the somatosensory cortex of the left cerebral hemisphere.

Visual information is consistently transmitted contralaterally. Information in the right visual field of each eye is transmitted to the left cerebral hemisphere. The reverse is true for the left visual field.

Auditory input is bilateral, each ear transmitting information to both sides of the brain. The majority of nerve fibers, however, cross to the auditory cortex opposite to the side of stimulation.

The major pathway for somatosensory information is contralateral, e.g., left body surface to right hemisphere, crossing at the brain stem. The secondary somatosensory pathway has some ipsilateral as well as contralateral connections.

**EFFERENT PATHWAYS.** The bulk of the efferent pathways similarly have contralateral representation in the brain. The majority of the pathways of the motor system cross at the level of the medulla as they leave the brain.

## REVIEW QUESTIONS

1. The basic unit of the nervous system is the neuron. True or False?
2. The axon receives nerve impulses. True or False?
3. Where does interneuronal communication take place?
4. Transmission of a nerve impulse involves the release and pickup of neurotransmitters. True or False?
5. The myelin sheath is made up of Golgi type I neurons. True or False?
6. What are the subdivisions of the peripheral nervous system?
7. What is the distinction between the posterior and anterior regions of the cerebral cortex?
8. Acetylcholine is a neurotransmitter. True or False?
9. What is the relationship between the central nervous system (CNS) and the autonomic nervous system (ANS)?
10. The spinal cord has two functions. What are they?
11. The Babinski sign is a pathological reflex. True or False?
12. The reticular activating system (RAS) is a substructure of the brain stem. True or False?
13. The cerebellum controls body balance and motor coordination. True or False?
14. What are the four lobes of the cerebral hemispheres and their functions?
15. Communication between the hemispheres is via the corpus callosum. True or False?

# 3

# TOPICS FOR SPECIAL CONSIDERATION: Brain Dysfunction, Critical Periods, Plasticity, Generalization from Adults to Children, Handedness, and Mental Retardation

There are several topics that are of particular importance in the study and practice of clinical child neuropsychology. Such topics derive their importance from either their prominent or controversial status in the current literature.

In this chapter we briefly discuss a selected sample of these topics: the term *brain dysfunction*, the concepts of critical periods and plasticity, difficulties in generalizing from adult data to children, handedness, and mental retardation.

## BRAIN DYSFUNCTION

*Brain dysfunction* is a term that refers to: (1) the structural, chemical, and/or biochemical abnormalities that occur in the brain; and (2) the consequences of such in-

FUNDAMENTALS OF CLINICAL CHILD NEUROPSYCHOLOGY

ISBN 0-8089-1910-5

**TABLE 3-1. REPRESENTATIVE DEVELOPMENTAL AND "PASTEL" CLASSIC SIGNS OF BRAIN DYSFUNCTION**

| DEVELOPMENTAL | "PASTEL" CLASSIC |
|---|---|
| Generalized clumsiness or slowness of fine motor and gross motor functions, e.g., difficulty holding a pencil, catching or throwing a ball | Lateralized or asymetric motor deficits, e.g., weakness on one side of the body |
| Bilateral overflow | Unilateral overflow |
| | Toe walking, broad-based gait |
| | Intention tremor |
| | Articulation errors, oromotor dyspraxia, drooling |

Adapted from Rapin, 1982.

sults in terms of brain functions. Recall that the brain comprises the cerebrum, the deep structures, the cerebellum, and the brain stem.

## Signs of Brain Dysfunction

The signs of brain dysfunction are traditionally divided into two classes: (1) the classic neurological signs and (2) the subtle signs.

The classic neurological signs are the manifestations of gross brain pathology. They include perceptual and sensory disorders, motor deficits, defects of cognitive and language functions, and seizure disorders. Emotional and behavioral disorders may also be the result of brain dysfunction.

The subtle deficits are often called "soft signs." Though relatively subtle compared to signs of gross brain pathology, they, too, affect a wide range of sensory, motor, and intellectual functions as well as emotions and behavior. For example, in a sensory function, a classic neurological sign of gross brain pathology is cortical blindness; a subtle sign is compromised visual analytic skills.

Some theorists have divided the "soft signs" into two groups: (1) the developmental and (2) the "pastel" classic. In the first group are a number of behavioral symptoms that do not necessarily reflect brain dysfunction but, rather, brain immaturity. These are considered abnormal behaviors when seen in older children but are normal for younger children and are sometimes outgrown. In contrast, the "pastel" signs are behaviors that are abnormal for a child of any age. These always reflect brain dysfunction. Table 3-1 presents a listing of representative developmental and "pastel" classic signs.

## Features of Brain Dysfunction

The consequences of brain insult depend upon: (1) the characteristics of the insult and (2) the characteristics of the individual who sustains it.

**CHARACTERISTICS OF THE INSULT.** Brain insult may be characterized by its extent and location. It may also be characterized as: diffuse or focal; structural, chemical, or biochemical; stable or progressive; acute or chronic; hereditary or acquired. Extent and location are probably the major determinants of the effects of cerebral insult on an individual's functioning.

**CHARACTERISTICS OF THE INDIVIDUAL.** An individual's functioning is the result of the interaction of genetic (intrinsic) and environmental (extrinsic) factors. The impact of both types of factors is felt throughout life. The features of brain dysfunction are determined by the interaction of genetic and environmental factors, as well as by certain characteristics of the individual. The principal variables are: (1) an individual's age at the time of onset of a brain disturbance, (2) his innate features, and (3) his life circumstances.

***Age.*** The nature and extent of the impact of brain insult is, in part, a function of the age or developmental stage at which it occurs. The concepts of critical periods and plasticity, discussed later in this chapter, are among the important factors that bear on this relationship.

***Innate Characteristics.*** The innate features of an individual, such as personality and intelligence, can impact significantly on the consequences of brain dysfunction. An individual's attitude toward his disorder, toward those who attempt to work with him, and toward the intervention strategies used, can influence the degree of success of attempts to ameliorate the consequences of the dysfunction.

An individual who is genetically endowed with high intelligence is often better able to develop compensatory mechanisms on his own. Intelligent individuals are often better able to learn and to generalize remedial techniques.

***Life Circumstances.*** Relevant life circumstances include one's environment, the presence or absence of supportive interpersonal relationships, and the diagnostic and treatment milieu.

## CRITICAL PERIODS

Critical periods in prenatal nervous system development are commonly defined as periods during which the organism is maximally sensitive to particular exogenous (external) influences. Most critical periods are paralleled by periods of rapid neurobiological growth or differentiation. During a critical period, certain factors, such as drugs or diseases, may seriously interfere with normal development.

The concept of postnatal critical periods is somewhat controversial. There is, however, evidence suggesting that there are critical periods for: (1) the growth of the central nervous system; (2) the growth of the visual pathways; (3) the formation of basic social relationships; and (4) the learning of language, cognitive, and motor skills.

## PLASTICITY

According to the concept of critical periods in brain development, the effects of insult are more profound on the developing brain than on the mature brain. There are two exceptions: (1) the younger, immature brain is less affected by hypoxia than the mature brain; and (2) the younger brain is less profoundly affected than the adult brain by certain forms of insult (e.g., trauma). The younger brain evidently has a greater recovery potential than the mature brain because of neuronal plasticity. In other words, during the time that neuronal tissue continues to differentiate, affected neurons may be replaced by new ones or by those recruited from an undifferentiated pool.

The consequences of insult to the more mature brain depend upon: (1) the extent to which the affected brain areas can recover and (2) the extent to which intact areas can take over their function. The recovery has been hypothesized to be based on: (1) the inherently redundant organization of the brain, (2) the functional reorganization potential of the brain, and (3) the development of new synaptic connections.

It has long been assumed that the brain's pliability is greater in childhood than in adulthood. This view is bolstered by the apparently greater ability of children to recover from early insult to the brain. For example, it is well known that dysfunction in the dominant hemisphere is more likely to produce more serious and permanent language disturbances in adults than in children.

Although it is recognized that the brain is able to recover from insult, it is also known that plasticity is limited, even in childhood. Some theorists, in fact, speculate that the resilience of the child's brain may be more apparent than real. For example, the effects of an early insult may not be evident at the time it occurs. The sequellae to the insult may emerge later, when more advanced functions that depend on the affected regions are expected to emerge.

## GENERALIZATION FROM ADULTS TO CHILDREN

As the study of developmental neuropsychology advances, it becomes more and more apparent that developmental syndromes of higher cortical dysfunction resemble those delineated in the adult population with acquired focal damage. Nevertheless, considerable caution should be exercised in generalizing from adults to children regarding brain-behavior relationships, since important differences do exist. For example:

1. Although the gross features of neonatal and adult brains are the same, the brain is immature at birth and undergoes considerable development thereafter. This development consists largely of increasing myelination of the neuronal pathways and development of the multiple and redundant neuronal interconnections that characterize the fully mature brain. The frequently described temporal sequence (four stages) of cortical development is schematically presented in Figure 3-1. Brain development also entails the increasing functional importance of certain structures, such as the corpus callosum, which are present at birth but probably not functional.

2. Damage to a fully developed adult brain usually affects behavior. In contrast, when there is early insult to brain regions whose functions are not yet developed, the effects of the resulting dysfunction are silent until that later time when behaviors

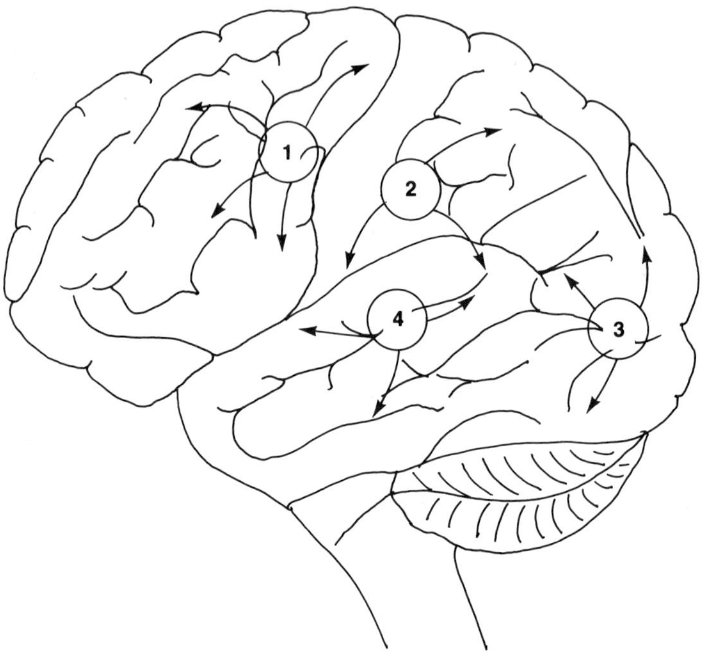


**Figure 3–1.** The frequently described temporal sequence of four stages of cortical development. (Adapted with permission from "Neurobiology of language" by H. A. Whitaker, in E. R. Carterette and M. P. Friedman (eds.): *Handbook of Perception*, vol. 7, Academic Press, 1976.)

**TABLE 3-2. A NUMBER OF MAJOR CAUSES OF BRAIN DYSFUNCTION IN CHILDREN AND ADULTS**

***Genetic***
Chromosomal disorders (e.g., Down syndrome)
Inherited disorders

***Unknown Prenatal Influences***
Hydrocephalus

***Gestation Disorders***
Prematurity
Low birth weight

***Infections***
Bacterial
Viral

***Toxins***
Endogenous (e.g., renal failure)
Exogenous (e.g., medicinal and illicit drugs)

***Metabolic Disorders***
Endocrine imbalance

***Nutrition***
Malnutrition

***Trauma***
Prenatal injury
Mechanical injury at birth
Perinatal hypoxia
Postnatal hypoxia
Postnatal injury

***Gross Brain Disease***
Cerebrovascular disorder

***Degenerative***
Alzheimer's disease

***Environmental Influences***
Severe psychosocial deprivation

dependent upon the region are expected to emerge. This makes it difficult not only to detect early insult to the brain in children but to know, in retrospect, whether an impairment in function is a reflection of early insult or of disturbed development.

3. The causes of brain dysfunction in adults are generally different from the causes of brain dysfunction in children. In adults, brain insult is usually focal. It is commonly the result of vascular events, tumors, or penetrating head injuries. In children, by contrast, brain insult is typically more generalized and less accessible to pathological diagnosis. Common causes are prenatal infections or chemical insults, perinatal trauma, intractable seizure disorders, or hereditary abnormalities. Table 3-2 lists a number of the major causes of brain dysfunction in children and adults.

4. The intellectual functioning of adults is different from that of children. Adults' functioning depends heavily on experience and on the ability to store and retrieve acquired information and integrate new information. Because children lack the store of previously acquired information possessed by adults, they focus the bulk of their intellectual efforts on new learning. The ability to learn, however, is frequently affected by brain dysfunction. As a consequence, if an adult and a child suffer comparable insult to the brain, the child may show more serious disorder than the adult. For example, if an adult and a young child each suffer insult to the receptive language region, the consequences for the adult will be limited to receptive language disorder. The child, still learning language skills, will manifest expressive as well as receptive language disturbances.

5. Changes in performance of adults and children on a test may have different meanings. Performance on a test can be conceptualized as the result of the interaction of three factors: (1) test behavior, e.g., motivation, distractibility; (2) social/cultural influences, e.g., school; and (3) underlying skill(s). For adults, test behavior and social/cultural influences are assumed to be constant over time and changes in test performance are assumed to be the consequence of changes in the underlying skill(s). With children, however, test behavior and social/cultural influences cannot be assumed to be comparable at different testings. For example, a child goes to school and is exposed to new experiences. Further, the same test does not measure the same skill(s) across age levels. Performance is influenced by the changing strategies of the developing child. An example of this is the influence of language on the performance of nonverbal tasks for some children as linguistic skills develop.

## HANDEDNESS

Interest in hand preference, an observable characteristic associated with language dominance, became popular in the 1920's. The interest grew out of the effort of investigators to study the relationship between cerebral dominance for language functions and cognitive performance.

Handedness is defined as either hand preference or as a difference between hands in skill level. Approximately 90 percent of all people are right-handed, 10 percent are left-handed. Left-handedness is considered to include ambidextrous individuals as well as those showing a clear preference for the left hand.

The relationship between handedness and the language-dominant hemisphere is well established. With few exceptions, right-handed individuals have language functions localized in the left cerebral hemisphere. Most left-handed people also have language functions localized in the left hemisphere. It is estimated that from 15 to 33 percent of left-handed individuals have right-lateralized language functions. A minority have some capacity for language in both hemispheres.

People are left-handed as the result of: (1) genetic diversity, (2) environmental factors, or (3) lateralized brain insult. Nonfamilial left-handedness may occur randomly. Such influence as social pressure or physical trauma to the right hand may cause a child who was genetically determined to be right-handed to be left-handed. Prenatal or perinatal damage to the left cerebral hemisphere may cause a shift of handedness. Left-handedness due to brain insult is called *pathological handedness.*

Handedness is assessed by: (1) preference or (2) difference between the two hands in performing manual tasks, such as writing and eating. Most children evidence consistent handedness by the age of six years.

Researchers have studied not only handedness, but consistency of "sidedness" and eyedness. This research has revealed no conclusive relationship between side preference and by inference cerebral dominance, and cognitive development.

## MENTAL RETARDATION

The term *mental retardation* refers to a general deficit in cognitive competence that results in failure to function adaptively. *Adaptive functioning* refers to the ability of an individual to meet the social and educational demands expected for his age and social group. Commonly used equivalent terms are *developmental handicap* and *mental deficiency.* It is estimated that approximately 1 percent of the child and adolescent population of the United States is mentally retarded.

The categories of mental retardation are based on deviation of general intellectual functioning from the average intelligence quotient (IQ) of 100. Assessment of general intellectual functioning is obtained through an individually administered general intelligence test. It is assumed that the individual is not suffering gross sensorimotor or emotional handicaps. The subtypes of mental retardation and IQ levels are:

| SUBTYPE OF MENTAL RETARDATION | IQ LEVEL |
|---|---|
| Mild | 50–70 |
| Moderate | 35–49 |
| Severe | 20–34 |
| Profound | Below 20 |

Mental retardation may be due to biological factors (e.g., CNS pathology), psychosocial factors (e.g., poor environmental conditions), or an interaction of both.

It is estimated that in approximately 25 percent of the cases, the etiology is known biological abnormalities. The most common are metabolic (e.g., phenylketonuria) and chromosomal (e.g., Down syndrome) disorders. In such cases the level of retardation is generally moderate to profound. Mental retardation due to biological abnormalities occurs with equal frequency across socioeconomic classes and is not more prevalent in other family members unless due to an underlying genetic disorder (e.g., Tay-Sachs disease).

Most cases of mental retardation are classified as mild, and commonly there is no known biological underlying factor. It is suggested that in these instances mental retardation exists due to an interaction of genetic endowment and poor environmental conditions. This was previously called cultural-familial retardation. The lower socioeconomic classes are over-represented in this group, and there is often a familial pattern of similar levels of mental retardation.

## REVIEW QUESTIONS

1. What makes up the brain?
2. Brain dysfunction always refers to structural abnormalities. True or False?
3. What is the difference between classic neurological signs and "soft signs"?
4. What are "pastel" classic signs?
5. The consequences of brain dysfunction depend upon what factors?
6. What are critical periods?
7. The younger brain has greater neuronal plasticity than the mature brain. True or False?
8. The plasticity of a child's brain is unlimited. True or False?
9. What are some reasons why caution must be exercised in generalizing from adults to children in the study of brain-behavior relationships?
10. Left-handed people have language lateralized to the right cerebral hemisphere. True or False?
11. What causes left-handedness?
12. Define mental retardation.
13. Mental retardation may be due to what factors?
14. What percentage of the population is right-handed?
15. Most cases of mental retardation are due to biological abnormalities. True or False?

# 4

# LANGUAGE AND SPEECH DISORDERS

Language and speech impact profoundly on a child's play, thinking processes, intellectual development, academic achievements, and emotional development. Through the mediation of language and speech, relationships with other people are formed and socialization takes place.

Questions about language or speech development or both are frequently the presenting concerns when a child is referred for an examination. Because language and speech play such a central role in a child's intellectual development and emotional well-being, language and speech functions should be assessed even when not questioned. Assessment of these functions is a central component of a comprehensive psychological evaluation.

In this chapter, we discuss the neuroanatomical basis of language and speech; define the clinical syndromes of language and speech disorders; summarize the requirements and timetable of language (including speech) development; discuss various models of developmental language disorders and childhood speech disorders that have been proposed; and present a guide to the diagnosis of language and speech disorders. Language disorders are discussed first.

## NEUROANATOMICAL BASIS OF LANGUAGE

The language process is often conceptualized as consisting of two main components: (1) the reception and (2) the expression of written and spoken language. Reception refers to: (1) the detection, (2) the discrimination, and (3) the interpretation of written and spoken symbols. The reception aspect of language processing is also

FUNDAMENTALS OF CLINICAL CHILD NEUROPSYCHOLOGY


ISBN 0-8089-1910-5

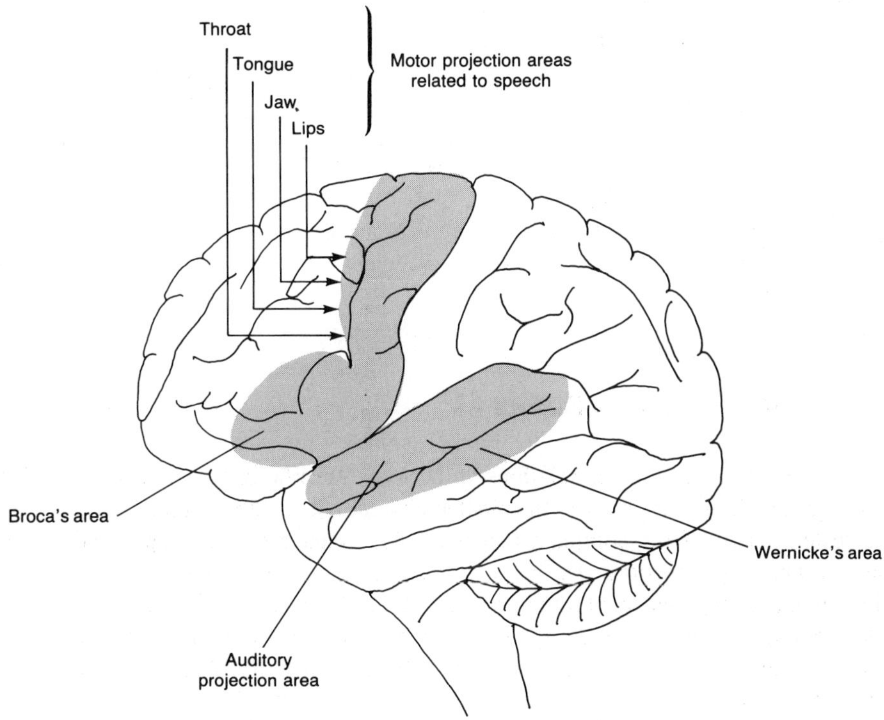


**Figure 4–1.** Projection and association areas most relevant to language functions. (Reproduced from *Psychology* by H. Gleitman by permission of W.W. Norton & Company, Inc. Copyright © 1981 by W.W. Norton & Company, Inc.)

referred to as *decoding*. Expression refers to the production of written or spoken symbols. The expressive aspect of language processing is also referred to as *encoding*.

Our knowledge of the neurological basis of language can be summarized as follows: We know that there are four regions of the dominant (usually left) hemisphere that play a crucial part in the reception (decoding) and expression (encoding) of language. Speech signals are transmitted through the auditory nerve and discriminated (decoded) in Heschl's gyrus, in the primary auditory area of the temporal lobe. The interpretation, or understanding of the meaning, of speech signals involves Wernicke's area, located in the posterior portion of the dominant (usually left) superior temporal gyrus. Broca's area, in the dominant inferior frontal gyrus, is responsible for the encoding of language. Verbalization is mediated by regions of the frontal lobe (Figure 4-1).

Specific and important aspects of linguistic activity (language-part functions) commonly associated with defined brain areas include:

1. Retention of sequential verbal material, associated with the inferior region of the dominant temporal lobe

2. Comprehension of logical grammatical relationships, associated with the dominant parietal-occipital and frontal regions
3. Appreciation of the rhythm of speech, associated with the posterior area of the right hemisphere
4. Repetition of speech words, associated with pathways in the dominant temporal or frontal speech areas and/or the pathways connecting these areas
5. Naming to visual confrontation, associated with the dominant temporal-parietal-occipital area and with Broca's area in the dominant frontal lobe
6. Expression of the rhythm of speech, associated with the anterior region of the right hemisphere

## ADULT LANGUAGE DISORDERS

Basic understanding of the relationship between specific brain regions and various language functions dates back to the nineteenth century. In 1861, Broca postulated that the posterior part of the dominant (usually left) frontal cortex is responsible for expressive language functions. He based this on results of his investigative work with adults who, having sustained structural damage to focal brain areas, suffered loss or deterioration of ability to speak (aphasia), to read (alexia) or to write (agraphia).

Today, the study of language disorders still relies heavily on the examination of adults with acquired brain dysfunction. Though there are admitted problems in extrapolating such data to children, this body of information is basic to understanding brain-behavior relationships as they apply to language functions in children. In the first place, it has enabled us to appreciate the fact that language is processed in a number of brain areas. Second, it has revealed the processing of language as a series of brain events that involves the decoding and encoding of information.

### Classification of Adult Language Disorders (Aphasias)

The adult aphasias may be divided into three categories: (1) the predominantly receptive, (2) the predominantly expressive, and (3) the receptive-expressive. These language disorders are grouped according to the presence or absence of a number of salient language functions. The definition and method of assessing these functions follow:

1. *Conversational speech*, which refers to an individual's spontaneous speech in conversation with the examiner. Spontaneous speech is assessed as fluent or dysfluent, based on the following criteria: amount of output, quality of articulation, quality of prosody (rhythm) of speech, presence of speech sound, syllable, or word substitutions.

2. *Comprehension*, which refers to an individual's understanding of spoken language. It is difficult to assess because comprehension depends upon nonlinguistic

functions (e.g., memory) as well as linguistic ones, and the tasks used to demonstrate comprehension typically utilize nonlanguage skills (e.g., the motor skills involved in speech and in responding to verbal commands). Further, comprehension ability is not an absolute (either present or absent).

Comprehension is assessed through quantitative measures and also through qualitative measures involving the systematic presentation of tasks graded in difficulty, beginning with simple pointing tasks and progressing to tasks that require the understanding of complex linguistic structures.

3. *Repetition*, which refers to the ability to accurately repeat information that is presented orally. Repetition ability is assessed through a variety of quantitative tasks, which typically involve repetition of an arbitrary series of numbers and words as well as meaningful sentences.

4. *Naming*, or word finding, difficulty, which is a feature common to all language disorders. The degree of severity, however, varies among language disordered individuals and among language disorder groups. In turn, there are a number of disorders other than language disorders in which naming difficulty is common (e.g., Alzheimer's disease). Thus, although difficulty in naming should always raise the question of a possible language disorder, it may, in fact, turn out to be a symptom of some other disease.

Naming difficulty may be apparent in spontaneous speech. It may be seen in: (1) failure to respond in a naming task, (2) use of neologisms (i.e., nonsense words or nonreal words), and (3) word substitutions. In addition, naming difficulty may be assessed directly through tasks involving confrontational naming (e.g., naming a visible object or color on demand).

5. *Reading*. Reading is a complex language skill that relies on a variety of language-based functions (e.g., auditory sequential memory) and nonlanguage-based functions (e.g., visual perception). A reading disorder, thus, may exist with or without a language disorder. Both oral reading and reading comprehension are assessed through quantitative and qualitative measures. Reading disorders are discussed in detail in Chapter 9.

6. *Writing*. An individual with a language disorder typically has a writing disorder as well. Writing is a complex task that is dependent upon the functioning of a number of brain systems, including those involved in language. A writing disorder can also exist in the absence of a language disorder, however. The full range of writing skills is assessed through quantitative and qualitative measures. Writing disorders are discussed in Chapter 10.

Principal features of the major adult aphasias are summarized in Table 4-1. Because a detailed delineation of the full range of adult aphasias is clearly beyond the scope of this book, we describe in some detail the symptom pattern of only one language disturbance in each of the three aphasia categories: namely, Wernicke's aphasia (predominantly receptive), Broca's aphasia (predominantly expressive) and conduction aphasia (receptive-expressive). We briefly note the main features of the other major adult aphasias.

**TABLE 4-1. PRINCIPAL FEATURES OF ADULT APHASIA**

| | Wernicke's | Broca's | Conduction | Anomic | Transcortical | | | Global |
|---|---|---|---|---|---|---|---|---|
| | | | | | *Sensory* | *Motor* | *Mixed* | |
| *Fluency* | + | - | + | + | + | - | - | - |
| *Comprehension of Oral Language* | - | + | + | + | - | + | - | - |
| *Repetition* | - | - | - | + | + | + | + | - |
| | | | | | ----- echolalia ----- | | | |
| *Naming* | - | - | - | - | - | - | - | - |
| *Reading Aloud* | - | - | - | + | + | + | - | - |
| *Reading Comprehension* | - | + | + | + | - | + | - | - |
| *Writing* | - | - | - | + | - | - | - | - |

+ Relatively spared
- Relatively impaired

### *Wernicke's Aphasia (Predominantly Receptive)*

In Wernicke's aphasia, also called sensory aphasia, an individual is fluent. There is no notable disturbance in either spontaneous speech production or articulation. Spontaneous speech consists of complete sentences with good syntactical and semantic value. Speech errors typically involve circumlocutions. Circumlocutions are convoluted ways of saying things. They are commonly used by individuals with word finding problems who tend to substitute words when they are unable to produce the one they need. Paraphasias (i.e., substitutions of words that are similar but that have different meaning) are common. In Wernicke's aphasia, the paraphasias typically consist of semantic substitutions (e.g., "timer" for "watch"). The cardinal features of this disorder are seriously impaired comprehension of oral language and very poor repetition ability. Naming ability is impaired and reading (both aloud and silently with comprehension) are also poor. Writing is always disturbed and commonly consists of letter combinations that look like real words but, in fact, are nonsense words.

Wernicke's aphasia most often involves the language-dominant (usually left) temporal lobe, particularly Wernicke's area, which is located in the left superior temporal gyrus. When the dysfunction is in the anterior portion of Wernicke's area, it affects word discrimination. Dysfunction in the posterior portion of Wernicke's area affects understanding of word meaning.

### *Broca's Aphasia (Predominantly Expressive)*

In Broca's aphasia, also called motor aphasia, an individual has difficulty producing speech sounds and is essentially nonfluent. Spontaneous speech is sparse. The phrases emitted are telegraphic and consist mostly of nouns and verbs. Articulation is poorest when the symbolic demands of speech are greatest but is intact when simple or automatic speech is required. Comprehension of oral language is relatively intact. Repetition and naming, however, are impaired. An individual with Broca's aphasia has very poor ability to read aloud. However, his ability to understand what he reads to himself is good. Typically, the ability to write is seriously disturbed.

An individual with Broca's aphasia usually has dysfunction in Broca's area, located in the inferior frontal gyrus of the language-dominant hemisphere.

### *Conduction Aphasia (Receptive-Expressive)*

An individual with conduction aphasia is fluent and has relatively normal comprehension of oral language. His speech is characterized by paraphasias, which are mostly of the literal variety (phonetic substitutions, e.g., "great" for "greed"). The cardinal feature of this aphasia is a serious disturbance in the ability to repeat words. Naming ability is, in addition, very poor, as is ability to read aloud. Though silent reading is unimpaired (as demonstrated in good reading comprehension), writing disturbances are common, if generally mild. Typically, writing problems involve reversals of words, letter insertions, or both.

Conduction aphasia has been associated with dysfunction in a variety of areas of the dominant temporal lobe.

### *Anomic, Transcortical, and Global Aphasias*

The main features of these adult aphasias are outlined below:

**ANOMIC APHASIA.** This syndrome is characterized by one notable disturbance, namely, a difficulty producing names on demand. The other salient language functions are intact. Anomic aphasia has been associated with dysfunction of both the language-dominant hemisphere and the nondominant hemisphere.

**TRANSCORTICAL SENSORY APHASIA.** This syndrome is characterized by intact fluency and intact ability to read aloud. Repetition functions are unimpaired and echolalia, the echoing of words that are spoken by another person, is common. Comprehension of oral language, naming ability, reading comprehension, and writing are all deficient. Transcortical sensory aphasia has been associated with dysfunction of the temporal and parietal regions and with the junction between these two areas.

**TRANSCORTICAL MOTOR APHASIA.** In this aphasia, comprehension of oral language is intact, as is the ability to read aloud and to understand what is read. Repetition ability is also spared. Echolalia is common. Naming and writing functions are disturbed. Fluency is markedly impaired. Transcortical motor aphasia has been associated with dysfunction in the dominant frontal lobe.

**TRANSCORTICAL MIXED APHASIA.** This syndrome is characterized by intact ability to repeat, which includes a tendency toward echolalia. There is serious disturbance in fluency, understanding of oral language, naming, reading aloud, understanding what is read, and writing. This disorder has been associated with the brain regions that surround Broca's area and Wernicke's area, and the cortical pathways connecting them.

**GLOBAL APHASIA.** This syndrome is characterized by a serious disturbance in all of the salient language functions. Global aphasia has been associated with dysfunction in Broca's and Wernicke's areas and in additional language regions of the dominant hemisphere.

## REQUIREMENTS OF LANGUAGE DEVELOPMENT

The normal development of language has been extensively studied. Although there are a number of highly respected theories of language development with quite different theoretical underpinnings (i.e., behavioral vs. neurolinguistic), there is no single comprehensive model of language development. Nevertheless, certain prerequisites to normal language development have been clearly defined. Generally speaking, the prerequisites of language acquisition can be divided into three groups: (1) biological, (2) environmental, and (3) psychological.

### Biological Prerequisites

In order to learn language skills a child must first of all possess adequate sensory acuity and adequate perceptual functions. In the case of a child learning auditory-verbal language, adequate auditory acuity, sound discrimination and phonemic discrimination are required. (With deaf children, sensory acuity and perceptual discrimination are similarly required for language acquisition. Because manual rather than verbal expression is used first, language acquisition by the deaf child also requires adequate levels of visual and somatosensory acuity and perception.) Language acquisition always depends upon brain areas that subserve memory or information storage. Expressive language depends upon brain areas that subserve certain motor functions.

Intellectual ability affects the rate at which language skills are mastered and the degree to which the ability to express complex ideas emerges. Language elaborations permit the expression of complex ideas. The mentally deficient are slower in learning language functions. While they eventually master the simple meanings of words and some rudimentary grammar rules for generating simple sentences, they fail to master language elaborations. For this reason, they remain limited in ability to express and comprehend the subtle nuances of language.

### Environmental Prerequisites

The quantity and quality of language to which a young child is exposed are also crucial to his language development. Acquisition of language is highly dependent on the presence of adequate language models. An adequate language model provides prelinguistic and verbal stimulation and communication. These require a minimal level of nonverbal and verbal interaction. A child with average intellectual potential may fail to develop language elaborations as a result of poor language models.

### Psychological Prerequisites

The acquisition of normal language requires the development of interpersonal relationships. The process begins at birth when the infant bonds to the mother. Later, it is seen in the prelinguistic infant who communicates with his caretakers by cooing, gesturing, babbling, and so on. This interaction establishes shared references to things and events in the environment and to emotions. Continued language development takes place within the context of emotional ties between the child and his language models. In the absence of age-appropriate related behavior, normal language fails to develop.

## TIMETABLE FOR LANGUAGE ACQUISITION

The development of language takes place within the framework of developing sensory/perceptual, motor and social skills. It involves a child's mastery of the phonology (speech sounds), syntax (grammar), and semantics (vocabulary) of his language environment. In addition, it depends upon his ability to use language pragmatically (in context).

By four to six years of age, without formal instruction, all normal children have acquired a high proficiency in their native language. The normal course of language acquisition and developing sensory/perceptual, motor and social skills is summarized in Table 4-2. Language acquisition is discussed below:

A newborn infant is able to discriminate individual speech sounds. An infant vocalizes from the first moment of life, beginning with crying. By around one month, he uses different sounds for pain and hunger.

By around two to three months of age, spontaneously produced sounds are referred to as babbling. Although these sounds have no real meaning, they do have a social quality. In other words, the cooing and babbling of an infant increase in the presence of a stimulating or responsive person. Prelinguistic communication also begins to emerge. The infant points to objects and gestures to communicate his wishes. Through this behavior, if successful, the infant begins to learn the communicative and referential functions of language.

At around four to six months, an infant "talks" to himself. Sounds are used to indicate pleasure and displeasure.

By about six to nine months of age, the infant can imitate speech sounds. This requires the ability to segment whole words into individual speech sound parts. Sounds that are not a part of a child's language experience drop out of his repertoire, and the sound parts of real whole words come to predominate. The infant responds to his name.

At about ten to twenty months, true speech begins to appear. The utterances are single words, typically referring to simple interactions (e.g., "bye-bye"), names, labels, adjectives, and verbs. Initially pointing, a child can nonverbally "label" objects and familiar people. The ability to use words depends upon a small child's skill in associating speech sounds with visual percepts. The child has a speaking vocabulary of five to fifty words.

At about the age of two to three years, a child begins to utter two- to three-word

**TABLE 4-2. TIMETABLE OF LANGUAGE, SENSORY/PERCEPTUAL, MOTOR AND SOCIAL SKILL DEVELOPMENT**

| AGE | LANGUAGE | SENSORY/PERCEPTUAL AND MOTOR | SOCIAL |
|---|---|---|---|
| Birth - 1 month | Cries, different sounds for pain and hunger | Sucks, swallows | |
| 2-3 months | Babbles, coos, prelinguistic communication begins | Physically responsive | Meaningful smile, prelinguistic communication begins |
| 4-6 months | "Talks" to self, different sounds for pleasure and displeasure | Turns toward sounds, gains in sitting posture, reaches for objects, picks up spoon | Laughs, responds to people during play, social smile |
| 6-9 months | Imitates speech sounds, puts sounds together and repeats, responds to name | Sits unassisted, recognizes familiar people and objects, grasps and pulls at things, drooling stops | Plays "peek-a-boo" and "patacake," pats image in mirror, waves "bye-bye" |
| 10-20 months | Single word utterances, understands gestures, responds to simple commands, speaking vocabulary of 5-50 words | Alerts visually to new objects, stands alone, walks unassisted, begins to feed self with spoon, marks with pencil, imitates 2-3 block tower | Interested in play with other people, pulls person to show things, shows or offers toys |
| 2-3 years | Makes 2-3 word phrases, syntax emerges, gives full name, identifies 5 objects, speaking vocabulary of about 300 words | Walks and runs well, goes up and down stairs unassisted, jumps, turns single pages of book, scribbles with pencil, imitates 3-4 block tower | Plays meaningfully with dolls, parallel play predominates, helps put things away, understands taking turns |
| 4 years | Understands basic rules of grammar, speaks in sentences, vocabulary of about 1000 words | Walks backward, imitates drawing of m and q, completes 8 piece form board | Associate play begins |
| 5-6 years | Language elaborations emerge, vocabulary expands | Imitates drawing of Δ | Associate play develops |

phrases. Systematic and meaningful, these utterances are the first evidence of emerging syntax, or grammar. By about two-and-a-half years of age, phrases consisting of several words begin to appear. By now, the child has a vocabulary of about three hundred words.

By about age four, a child is able to demonstrate the basic rules of grammar by producing grammatically correct sentences. The factors underlying the grammatical aspect of language development and the manner in which grammatical skills are perfected as they evolve are very poorly understood. This remains a topic of great interest and debate. The child now has a vocabulary of about one thousand words.

By about five to six years of age, the ability to abstract and generalize develops, and verbs, adjectives, and relational words are added to a child's vocabulary. More refined language elaborations soon emerge; these include functor words such as *and* and *but*, and morphemes (changes in word structure that alter word meaning, such as the addition of the endings *-ed* or *-ing*, which permit the creation of complex propositions). Vocabulary expands (to about two thousand words or more).

Unlike the early acquisition of oral language, which proceeds without formal instruction, the later acquisition of written language skills, namely reading, writing, and arithmetic, requires a great deal of teaching and practice. Reading, writing, and arithmetic are special language skills in and of themselves. In addition, they depend heavily on a broad range of language subskills. A discussion of the relation between language and language subskills and the learning of reading, writing, and arithmetic is presented in Chapters 9, 10, and 11, respectively.

## CHILDHOOD LANGUAGE DISORDERS

Language disturbances in children can be divided into two general categories: (1) acquired disturbances and (2) developmental disturbances.

An acquired language disturbance is an impairment (or loss) of normal language resulting from a brain dysfunction that occurs after language has developed. Two-and-one-half years is the delineating age. Acquired language disturbance in children, as in adults, is called aphasia.

A developmental language disturbance (dysphasia) may be manifested by failure to develop language, delay in language acquisition, or development of deviant language. Dysphasia is not the result of an acquired brain dysfunction.

### Acquired Language Disorders

Despite the fact that children with acquired language disturbances are a very small minority of those who suffer from deficient language ability, the literature tends to focus upon this type of disorder.

The classification system used for aphasia in adults is typically applied to childhood aphasia. Thus, children with acquired language disturbances are classified on the basis of having: (1) predominantly receptive, (2) predominantly expressive or, (3) receptive-expressive aphasia.

### Developmental Language Disorders

In the majority of language-disabled children, the disorder is of the developmental variety, referred to as dysphasia. To date, there is no agreed-upon classification of developmental language disturbances. Hence they are defined operationally and commonly identified by exclusion. Typically, this is accomplished through the use of some combination of the following criteria:

1. A language disturbance that exists in the absence of any severe psychological disturbance
2. A language disturbance that exists in the absence of serious environmental deprivation
3. A language disturbance that exists within the context of adequate intellectual potential

4. The presence of a verbal I.Q. that is 12 to 15 points lower than a performance I.Q.
5. Performance on a standardized test of language functions that is two years below the age-expected level or more than one standard deviation below the norm
6. Absence of any known cerebral injury

## MODELS OF DEVELOPMENTAL LANGUAGE DISORDERS

A variety of models of developmental language disturbances have been proposed. These can be divided into two groups: (1) the neuropsychological and (2) the neurolinguistic.

### Neuropsychological

Neuropsychological models are based on the assumption that the brain-behavior relationships in language disorders, both acquired and developmental, are the same in children and in adults. Additionally, in these models there is an implicit recognition of the universal presence of expressive disturbances in childhood disorders. Thus, the term *receptive* disturbance refers, in children, to symptom patterns in which there is a relatively more severe difficulty in comprehension than in verbal production.

There are two basic neuropsychological models. One model defines the disturbances as either receptive or expressive. The other model subdivides the disturbances into three categories: (1) receptive, (2) central processing, and (3) expressive. In the first model, it is assumed that a language disorder reflects a specific deficit in either language reception or language expression. In the second, this view of receptive and expressive disorders is accepted, but it is further suggested that deficits in central processing also occur. This latter category consists of defects in comprehension that exist in the presence of unimpaired reception and expression of language. The precise nature of central processing disorders remains poorly defined.

### Neurolinguistic

The neurolinguistic models of developmental language disorders represent an attempt to classify language disturbances on the basis of symptom complexes without making any assumptions about neurological underpinnings. Some examples of the types of syndromes included in such models are:

**SEMANTIC-PRAGMATIC SYNDROME.** This syndrome is characterized by poor comprehension. Phonological decoding and encoding are unimpaired. Fluency is good. Anomia is common. There is poor pragmatic use of language.

**COMPREHENSION-PHONOLOGICAL SYNDROME.** This syndrome is characterized by poor comprehension plus poor speech.

**SEVERE EXPRESSIVE SYNDROME.** In this pattern, there is good comprehension but no speech.

**VERBAL AUDITORY AGNOSIA.** This syndrome is characterized by poor phonological decoding, which precludes development of normal speech. Language that is visually presented can be processed normally. This syndrome must be carefully differentiated from deafness.

**PHONOLOGICAL-SYNTACTICAL SYNDROME.** This pattern is characterized by very poor speech. Problems with articulation, syntax, and anomia are generally present. Comprehension is variable but is always better than expression.

## DIAGNOSIS OF LANGUAGE DISORDERS

The diagnosis of language disorders involves a determination of: (1) whether or not a language problem exists and (2) the relationship between language and nonlanguage functions, if a language disorder is identified. The latter task, which is very difficult, involves a determination of the extent to which a nonlanguage (behavioral, cognitive, or emotional disorder) is secondary to a language disorder or vice versa.

Language is an extremely complex neurological function, which affects and is affected by essentially all aspects of an individual's state, including his intellect, thinking processes, academic achievement, emotional well-being, and environmental situation. Some disturbances appear as primary language problems when in fact they are features of some other disorder (e.g., autism, retardation). On the other hand, a primary language disturbance may be obscured by some other specific learning disturbance (e.g., a reading or arithmetic disorder). It is only through a systematic and comprehensive evaluation that a psychologist can make an appropriate differential diagnosis of the presenting problem.

The most important differential diagnoses in the language area are between language disorders and the following:

1. Peripheral hearing loss or central deafness
2. Defective speech organ physiology
3. Severe environmental (including psychological, physical, and emotional) deprivation
4. Pervasive developmental disorder (e.g., childhood autism)
5. Childhood psychosis
6. Nonpsychotic behavioral disorder
7. Mental retardation
8. Severe memory disorder
9. Nonlanguage based reading and writing disturbance
10. Normal variation in language development

The differential diagnosis of a language disorder depends upon the combined efforts of specialists in audiology and speech and language pathology. The role of the psychologist is to: (1) make a preliminary delineation of a child's language functions and (2) make appropriate referrals to audiologists and speech and language specialists when a significant speech/language disorder is suspected or clearly revealed.

## Assessment of Language Competence and Language Subskills

An assessment of a child's language functions and language subskills requires the integration of quantitative and qualitative information. Quantitative measures are derived from a child's performance on standardized tests of language competence and subskills. Qualitative information is obtained from many different sources (e.g., reports from parents and teachers, special clinical procedures). A summary of representative assessment measures of language functions and subskills is presented in Appendix 5.

### *Quantitative Measures*

**LANGUAGE COMPETENCE.** The major standardized tests of global verbal competence are the intelligence tests. They provide a verbal intelligence score. Because these tests were not designed to assess language functions per se, it is possible to obtain a high verbal intelligence score and, at the same time, have a language disorder. Similarly, a low verbal score provides inadequate evidence of a language problem. Thus, significant language disorders may escape detection or remain poorly defined whenever the psychologist relies solely upon results of intelligence tests in assessing a child's language competence. Standardized tests specifically designed to assess receptive and expressive language functions are available and should be used.

**LANGUAGE SUBSKILLS.** Two classes of language subskills must be evaluated in assessing a child's language functions. The first includes all of the specific features of language described earlier (e.g., fluency, naming). The second includes the neuropsychological functions that underlie a child's ability to master language (e.g., auditory discrimination, auditory memory, and articulation skills). There are numerous standardized measures of language subskills.

### *Qualitative Measures*

The qualitative assessment of a child's language functions utilizes data obtained from an interview with the parent (or guardian), from school reports, and from clinical observation of the child. Common emotional and behavioral characteristics of children with language disorders are summarized in Table 4-3.

**PARENT (GUARDIAN) INTERVIEW.** Information is obtained about a child's language development and current language skills. The distinction between speech and language is stressed. A description of a child's language and speech is obtained.

In addition to a developmental history, the psychologist obtains medical and family histories; familial patterns of language and speech disturbances are noted (see Appendix 2).

**SCHOOL REPORT.** The school report provides information about a child's

**TABLE 4-3. COMMON BEHAVIORAL AND EMOTIONAL CHARACTERISTICS OF CHILDREN WITH LANGUAGE DISORDERS**

| |
|---|
| **BEHAVIORAL** |
| Minimal use of language |
| Evidence of deviant language/speech patterns |
| Use of gestures and/or drawings for self-expression |
| Difficulty understanding |
| Disruptive or abnormal behavior or both |
| Less than expected level of academic achievement |
| Poor work habits |
| Lack of work motivation |
| Social immaturity |
| Fine or gross motor impairment or both |
| Poor memory skills |
| **EMOTIONAL** |
| Anxiety |
| Depression |
| Disobedient, negativistic, and provocative behavior |
| Antisocial behavior |
| Developmentally inappropriate inattention and impulsivity, with or without a pattern of haphazard, poorly organized, non-goal-directed motor activity |

language-based academic achievements and his effective use of language as revealed in class participation (see Appendix 3).

**CLINICAL OBSERVATION.** Clinical observation provides information about the quality of a child's performance: (1) on standardized tests of language functions, (2) on age-appropriate tests of language functions, and (3) in spontaneous language functions. This information is vital to a delineation of a child's language functions. The quality of both receptive and expressive functions should be noted. The difference between spontaneous and responsive expressive skills should also be noted (see Appendix 4).

## SPEECH DISORDERS

Disordered speech occurs with significant frequency among the child population referred for psychological evaluation. It is the task of the psychologist to identify aberrant speech patterns and to begin to tease apart the possible underlying causes of speech problems. This requires an appreciation of the neuroanatomical basis of speech and of the behavior patterns that characterize each of the clinical speech disorder syndromes.

### Neuroanatomical Basis of Speech

A detailed description of the neuroanatomical basis of speech is not within the scope of this book. For our purposes, suffice it to say that competent speech depends upon: (1) the peripheral nerves, (2) the auditory and somatosensory cortex, (3) the frontal (motor) area of the cerebral cortex, and the systems that subserve motor

**TABLE 4-4. SPEECH DISORDER SYNDROMES**

I. Language-related disorders
II. Articulation disorders
III. Apraxic speech disorders
IV. Fluency disorders
V. Voice disorders

functions, (4) Wernicke's area in the dominant superior temporal gyrus, (5) Broca's area in the dominant inferior frontal gyrus, and (6) the connections between Wernicke's and Broca's areas and the motor cortex.

## Clinical Speech Disorder Syndromes

There are many types of speech disorders. The five most frequently seen by a psychologist are: (1) language-related speech disorders, (2) articulation disorders, (3) apraxic speech disorders, (4) fluency disorders, and (5) voice disorders. Language-related speech disorders and apraxia are always associated with neurological dysfunction. Articulation disorders, fluency disorders, and voice disorders may or may not be associated with neurological dysfunction. The speech disorder syndromes are summarized in Table 4-4 and discussed below.

### *Language-Related Disorders*

In language-related speech disorders, there is a disturbance in the ability to use speech as a symbolic tool. In these disorders, speech is characterized by a paucity of output and by telegraphic phrases. Articulation deteriorates in proportion to the symbolic content of the attempted speech. Automatic speech (e.g., the number sequence) is not affected. There are errors of omission. There may be errors of grammar and of word usage. Substitutions of speech sounds, syllables, and words are common.

Speech disorders associated with language disturbances reflect dysfunction in Broca's area.

### *Articulation Disorders*

Articulation errors occur commonly in the course of speech acquisition and have been found to follow specific patterns. Typically, however, children are able to master articulation of all the phonemes by approximately six years of age. A child who fails to do this may have an articulation disorder.

Articulation disorders are characterized by deviant production of speech sounds. Articulation errors may include substitutions and omissions in production of the phonemic elements of speech.

In articulation disorders, the underlying problem is commonly associated with dysfunction in the peripheral nerves, the motor cortex or motor systems, or structures that are crucial to articulation (e.g., the tongue).

### *Apraxic Speech Disorders*

Apraxic speech disorders are characterized by a disturbance in the motor programming aspect of speech. They may involve a poor ability to initiate nonverbal as well as verbal movements of the speech musculature (e.g., sticking out the tongue, opening and closing the jaw). In such cases, the disturbance is referred to as oromotor apraxia. When the disturbance is limited to verbal movements, it is called verbal apraxia.

Articulation errors in verbal apraxia are different from those seen in articulation disorders. They are inconsistent (not readily predictable). In addition, they are usually substitution errors, not sound distortion errors; and they are apparent in purposeful, but not in automatic speech.

Though often seen concurrently with Broca's aphasia, apraxic speech disorders must be regarded as distinct clinical entities.

Apraxic speech disorders are associated with dysfunction of a small region of Broca's area.

### *Fluency Disorders*

Fluency disorders are a disturbance in the prosody of speech.

In disorders of fluency, commonly referred to as stuttering, speech patterns are characterized by the repetition or prolongation of sounds, syllables, or words. Long pauses (or "blocks") often occur. The child who stutters typically experiences stress and anxiety around his dysfluency. He may develop a pattern of avoiding situations in which he is likely to have to speak.

Young children are often dysfluent, and such dysfluency is commonly considered to be a part of the normal developmental sequence of speech acquisition. Persistence of dysfluency beyond six years of age, however, is commonly defined as a speech disorder.

There is no one accepted explanation for stuttering. Current explanations come from learning theory, psychoanalytical theory, and our understanding of brain-behavior relations.

### *Voice Disorders*

Voice disorders are clinically defined as disturbances in an individual's voice that affect its quality (e.g., hoarseness), loudness, pitch (e.g., too high, monopitch), or all three. The sudden changes in pitch that occur in boys during puberty are frequently referred to as transient voice disorders.

Disturbances in voice may be associated with neurological dysfunction or with functional causes (e.g., hearing loss, emotional disorder).

## Speech Disorders in Children

Consistent with the general differences between adults and children with respect to brain dysfunction and level of speech experience (or amount of practice), speech disorders in children tend to be more subtle than those in adults. Developmental factors must be considered whenever a speech disorder is suspected in a child.

## Diagnosis of Speech Disorders

The diagnosis of a speech disorder is accomplished through the combined efforts of the psychologist, audiologist, and speech and language pathologist. When a child presents with a speech problem, the major task before the psychologist is to: (1) make a preliminary assessment of his speech functions and (2) determine whether or not the speech problem is a reflection of a language disorder. This involves use of standardized measures of both language and speech functions (summarized in Appendix 5). Qualitative assessment of speech depends upon the psychologist's careful attention to a child's verbalizations on standardized tests, on age-appropriate tasks, and in spontaneous conversation.

Whenever a child presents with a significant speech disorder, he is referred to an audiologist, and/or a speech and language specialist for further evaluation.

# REVIEW QUESTIONS

1. In which principal brain region is Broca's area located?
2. What is the main difference between aphasia and dysphasia?
3. What aspect of language processing depends upon the primary auditory receiving of the cortex?
4. Where in the brain is the primary auditory receiving area?
5. What language function does Wenicke's area subserve?
6. Language-dependent functions depend solely upon the left hemisphere. True or False?
7. Language development is a passive process. True or False?
8. Most children with language disorders have acquired brain dysfunction. True or False?
9. All speech disturbances reflect language disturbances. True or False?
10. What is the neuroanatomical basis of speech?
11. What is the single most prominent feature of acquired language disorders in children?
12. Reading and language disorders in children are not related. True or False?
13. What are the principle feature of conduction aphasia?
14. All children who fail to develop speech have severe language disorders. True or False?
15. Articulation errors are always an indication of an articulation disorder. True or False?

# 5

# EPISODIC DISORDERS: Epileptic Seizure Disorders, Seizure Disorders of Infancy and Childhood, and Headaches

Episodic disorders are characterized by a series of distinct and separate events that occur over time. An overview of three episodic disorders, epileptic seizures, seizures of childhood, and headaches, is presented in this chapter. Epileptic seizure disorders are discussed first.

## EPILEPTIC SEIZURE DISORDERS

The diagnosis and treatment of epileptic seizure disorders are the province of the neurologist. Nevertheless, the psychologist working with children must have considerable knowledge of these disorders for a number of reasons.

First, epileptic seizure disorders occur in children with relative frequency. Epidemiological studies have reported that they occur in as many as 5 out of every 100 individuals and that approximately 90 percent of all individuals with epileptic seizure disorders develop their initial symptoms before the age of twenty. Because the chance is great that the psychologist will be called upon to evaluate a child who has an undiagnosed epileptic seizure disorder, he must be aware of the range of the possible symptoms of these disorders. When such symptoms are recognized, a referral to a neurologist for medical evaluation is necessary.

FUNDAMENTALS OF CLINICAL CHILD NEUROPSYCHOLOGY


ISBN 0-8089-1910-5

**TABLE 5-1. CLASSIFICATION OF EPILEPTIC SEIZURE DISORDERS**

| |
|---|
| **PARTIAL (OR FOCAL) SEIZURES** |
| Simple partial seizures (consciousness not impaired)* |
| Complex partial seizures (consciousness impaired)* |
| Partial seizures that evolve to generalized seizures* |
| **GENERALIZED SEIZURES (CONSCIOUSNESS ALWAYS IMPAIRED)** |
| Absence (petit mal) seizures* |
| Myoclonic seizures |
| Clonic seizures |
| Tonic seizures |
| Tonic-clonic (grand mal) seizures* |
| Atonic seizures |
| **UNCLASSIFIED SEIZURES** |

*Seizures most often occurring in children.

Second, epileptic disorders can impact on a child's intellectual and cognitive functioning and emotional well-being. The assessment of these areas is the classical province of psychologists. Called upon to do a differential diagnosis of a child's learning, emotional, and behavioral problems, the psychologist must be knowledgeable about the potential effect of epileptic seizure disorders on a child's growth and development in a number of areas and on a child's performance on the tests used to assess higher cortical functions and personality development.

In this section we present an introduction to epileptic seizure disorders. We define epileptic seizure phenomena; outline the types of disorders that most frequently occur in children; summarize the relationship between epileptic disorders and intellectual functioning and personality; discuss the etiology of epileptic seizure disorders; present an overview of diagnostic procedures and treatment; and describe the role of the psychologist in the diagnostic process.

## Definition of Epileptic Seizure Disorders and Commonly Used Descriptive Terms

Epileptic seizures are the result of paroxysmal alterations in neuronal activity in the brain during which the neuronal discharges become abnormal and uncontrolled. The abnormal neuronal discharges are manifested clinically in episodic disturbances of consciousness, language, cognition, affect, sensory experience, and behavior, which an individual typically experiences as unpleasant (e.g., a noxious odor). The nature of the clinical manifestation of the seizure is a function of the site of the abnormal discharges.

An individual who experiences recurrent epileptic seizures is usually diagnosed as having epilepsy.

Interictal interval refers to the period of time between two epileptic seizures.

The period after an epileptic seizure is called the postictal period.

The seizure period itself is called the intraictal period.

When epileptic seizures occur one after the other without intervening consciousness, the condition is called status epilepticus. It requires immediate medical attention.

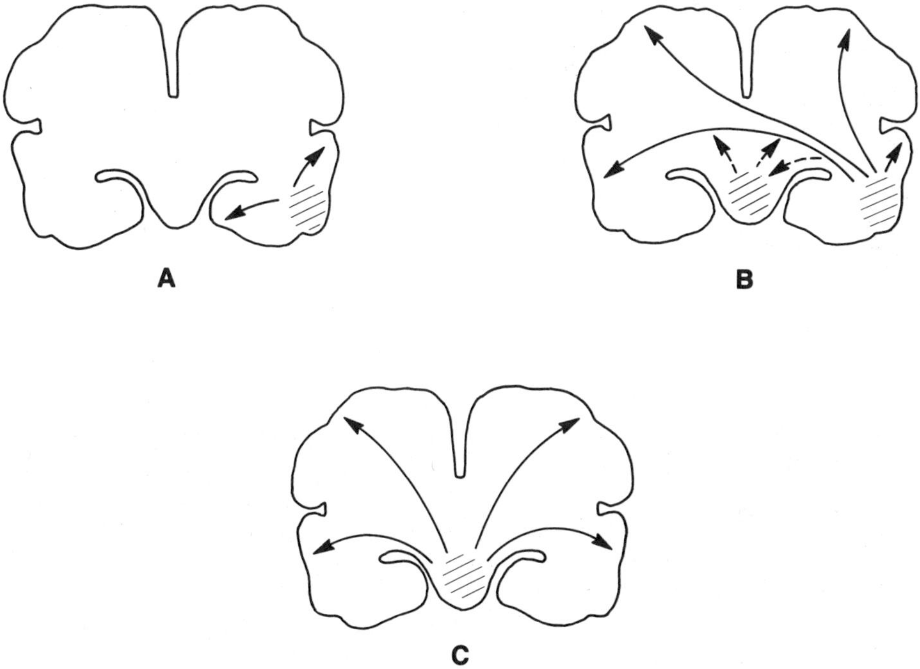


**Figure 5–1.** Spread of bioelectrical activity associated with types of epileptic seizures: *A*. Partial (or focal) seizures; *B*. Partial seizures that secondarily generalize; *C*. Primarily generalized seizures. (Adapted with permission from *Zerebrale anfalle im Kindesalter* by H. Doose. Desitin, 1975.)

## Types of Epileptic Seizure Disorders

There are two main categories of epileptic seizures: (1) partial (or focal) and (2) generalized. Partial seizures are localized to a part of the cerebral cortex or to a subcortical region; secondary generalization may occur if focal seizure activity spreads to the entire cortex. Primary generalized epileptic seizures, by contrast, are thought to begin in the brain stem, spreading to involve the whole cortex from the start. The patterns of abnormal electrical activity associated with the various types of epileptic seizures are presented in Figure 5-1.

Table 5-1 summarizes the classification of epileptic seizure disorders.

### *Partial (or Focal) Seizures*

Partial (or focal) seizures can develop in children or adults and are divided into three groups: (1) partial seizures with elementary (or simple) symptoms, (2) partial seizures with complex symptoms, and (3) partial seizures that become secondarily generalized.

**SIMPLE PARTIAL SEIZURES.** In simple partial epileptic seizures, consciousness

**TABLE 5-2. DIFFERENCES BETWEEN COMPLEX PARTIAL SEIZURES MANIFESTED SOLELY BY IMPAIRED CONSCIOUSNESS AND PETIT MAL SEIZURES**

| FEATURE | COMPLEX PARTIAL SEIZURE | PETIT MAL SEIZURE |
|---|---|---|
| ***Age of Onset*** | Any age | Childhood |
| ***Aura*** | Yes | No |
| ***Duration*** | Minutes | Seconds |
| ***Frequency*** | Few per day or less | May be many per day |
| ***Precipitants*** | No | Hyperventilation |
| ***Postictal Confusion*** | Yes | No |

Adapted from Cummings, 1985.

is not impaired. These seizures may be manifested by psychic, autonomic, sensory, and motor symptomology. Psychic symptoms may be manifested by language disorders, cognitive distortion, and affective sensations. Autonomic disturbances (e.g., flushing, pallor) may occur. Sensory symptoms commonly involve somatosensory, visual, auditory, gustatory (taste), olfactory, or vertiginous (unbalanced) sensations. An epileptic seizure that triggers an olfactory hallucination is often called an uncinate seizure or fit. Partial (or focal) seizures with motor symptoms were formerly called focal motor seizures. They involve rhythmic jerking of one area of the body, called clonic movements. Such a seizure may spread to half an individual's body, in which case it is referred to as a Jacksonian march.

**COMPLEX PARTIAL SEIZURES.** Complex partial seizures are epileptic seizures with complex symptomology. Consciousness is always affected to some degree. Psychic, autonomic, psychosensory, and psychomotor disturbances may occur. Complex partial seizures are also called temporal lobe seizures or psychomotor seizures, although the anatomical focus of the seizures may not be in the temporal lobe and psychomotor automatisms may not be part of the symptomology.

In the simplest type of complex partial seizure, only consciousness is affected for a brief period of time. There are no other symptoms. These brief lapses of consciousness are sometimes misdiagnosed as petit mal seizures, discussed below. A number of differences between these two types of seizure disorders are summarized in Table 5-2. Psychic manifestations of complex partial seizures may include intellectual symptomology. Language disorders may occur. Cognitive functioning may be affected. There may be memory distortion. In the phenomenon of *déja vu*, an individual feels that he is reliving an experience. In its counterpart, *jamais vu*, familiar people or objects appear novel. Intellectual rumination, also referred to as *forced thinking*, or *thought blocking*, may be experienced. Some individuals report feeling strong emotions, such as fear or depression. Autonomic disturbances may occur. Psychosensory symptoms are also reported. Visual disturbances occur frequently. Objects and people may appear too small (microscopia), too large (macroscopia), or misshapen (metamorphosia). Whole scenes recalling personal events may be envisioned. Auditory hallucinations are typically characterized by familiar voices repeating the

**TABLE 5-3. REPRESENTATIVE PSYCHOMOTOR AUTOMATISMS**

| |
|---|
| **SIMPLE PSYCHOMOTOR AUTOMATISMS** |
| Incoordination |
| Pushing |
| Chewing |
| Lip smacking |
| Groping |
| Swallowing |
| Staring |
| Spitting |
| Plucking |
| **SPEECH AUTOMATISMS** |
| Shouting |
| Screaming |
| Verbal reiteration |
| **AFFECTIVE AUTOMATISMS** |
| Gelastic epilepsy (laughing) |
| Dacrystic epilepsy (crying) |
| **COMPLEX AUTOMATISMS** |
| Cursive epilepsy (running) |
| Drinking |
| Prolonged twilight states with automatisms |
| Primitive masturbation |
| Undressing |

Adapted from Cummings, 1985.

same word or sound. Olfactory hallucinations are also common in complex partial seizures.

The behavioral abnormalities that typically occur in complex partial seizures consist of psychomotor automatisms. These are simple, habitual movements that are performed repeatedly (perseveration) and purposelessly (e.g., picking at one's clothes, turning one's head to one side). More complex automatisms, such as removal of clothing, rarely occur. Directed, violent behavior rarely occurs as a manifestation of a complex partial seizure. Examples of psychomotor automatisms are presented in Table 5-3.

During the postictal period following a complex partial seizure, an individual usually experiences a slow clearing of consciousness. He may become agitated during this period or he may experience euphoria. Language and speech disturbance may also occur. The disruption of behavior may be so severe that an individual is said to be experiencing postictal psychosis.

**PARTIAL SEIZURES THAT SECONDARILY GENERALIZE.** A partial (or focal) seizure may secondarily generalize to involve the whole cortex. The generalized seizure is usually a tonic-clonic seizure (discussed below). This is thought to occur when focal seizure activity in the cortex spreads to a subcortical pacemaker, such as the reticular activating system (RAS), which in turn spreads seizure activity throughout the cortex. Seizure activity may also spread across hemispheres via the commissures. The symptom of a focal seizure (e.g., olfactory hallucination) experienced prior to secondary generalization is called an aura.

**TABLE 5-4. DIFFERENCES BETWEEN PSYCHOMOTOR SEIZURES AND PSYCHOTIC BEHAVIOR**

| FEATURE | SEIZURE | PSYCHOSIS |
|---|---|---|
| ***Onset*** | Sudden (minutes) | Gradual (hours to days) |
| ***Duration*** | Minutes to hours | Several hours to days |
| ***Aura*** | May be | No |
| ***Contact with Environment*** | Tenuous and fluctuating | Tenuous and fluctuating to continual |
| ***Motor Activity*** | Automatisms; violence rare | May be complex, purposeful; agitation and violence possible |
| ***Intellectual Ability*** | Impaired | May be intact, but agitation or hallucinations interfere |
| ***Speech*** | May be dysarthric or aphasic | May be pressured or mute |
| ***Hallucinations*** | Stereotyped hallucinations or entire scenes viewed passively | Usually auditory of varied content, often interacted with |
| ***Conclusion*** | Gradual, with residual confusion | Gradual |
| ***Recollections of Episode*** | Variable | Yes |

Adapted from Kaufman, 1981.

### *Generalized Seizures*

In generalized seizures, consciousness is lost. Absence (petit mal) and tonic-clonic (grand mal) seizures are the generalized seizure disorders that most frequently occur in children.

**ABSENCE.** Simple absences, or petit mal seizures, consist of brief periods of loss of consciousness which may last for one to ten seconds. They may occur frequently, sometimes as often as dozens of times a day. Because the symptomology is so subtle, absences can go entirely undetected. An individual having an absence appears to be staring blankly into space. This is often mistaken for daydreaming. Absences may be confused with the simplest type of complex partial seizure (see Table 5-2). In complex absences, simple automatisms occur; for example, sucking motions. Muscles of the face, eyelids, and extremities may show subtle movement. During an absence, an individual will not respond to the environment. When the absence is over, he typically has no memory of the episode. He resumes activities quickly, having no postictal drowsiness or confusion.

Absences usually first occur between the ages of four and ten years but may begin in adolescence. They tend to disappear in early adulthood. In about half the cases of children who experience absences, a grand mal seizure disorder develops later.

**TONIC-CLONIC.** Tonic-clonic, or grand mal, seizures are a type of generalized seizure in which consciousness is lost and violent motor activity occurs. The motor activity is in two phases. In the first phase an individual's muscles become rigid. Since the rigidity makes it impossible to maintain posture, he falls. Contractions of the diaphragm and chest muscles may produce a shrill scream, called the epileptic cry. After the tonic phase, the clonic phase emerges. In the clonic phase, rhythmic contractions of the muscles shake the body violently. The contractions become gradually less frequent and less intense. During this phase, there may be vomiting and/or emptying of the bowel and bladder. In the postictal period of a grand mal seizure, an individual is unresponsive to his environment and his muscles are flaccid. He may fall asleep. If he

**TABLE 5-5. DIFFERENCES BETWEEN TONIC-CLONIC (GRAND MAL) SEIZURES AND PSEUDOEPILEPTIC SEIZURES**

| FEATURE | TONIC-CLONIC | PSEUDOEPILEPTIC |
|---|---|---|
| ***Onset*** | Abrupt | Often gradual |
| ***Body Movements*** | Rigidity, then tonic-clonic | Struggling, asynchronous |
| ***Biting*** | Tongue | Lips, arms, other areas of the body |
| ***Self-Injury*** | Common | Rare |
| ***Postictal Confusion*** | Present | Absent |
| ***Consciousness*** | Lost | Complete or partial |
| ***Duration*** | 30 seconds to a few minutes | Several to many minutes |
| ***Initiation or termination by suggestion*** | No | Yes |

Adapted from Cummings, 1985.

is awakened from this sleep, he is usually confused. The individual has no memory of the seizure episode.

## Personality, Intelligence, and Epileptic Seizure Disorders

Questions regarding the relationship between seizure disorders, personality, and intellectual functioning focus on two issues: (1) the differentiation of emotional and epileptic seizure disorders and (2) the impact of a seizure disorder on an individual's personality and intellectual functioning.

### *Differentiation of Emotional and Seizure Disorders*

The question of the difference between sensory experiences and abnormal behaviors due to a severe emotional disturbance and those due to a seizure disorder is most often raised regarding psychomotor seizures. During such seizure episodes, an individual may experience a wide variety of language, cognitive, affective, sensory, and behavioral disturbances. These symptoms may lead to the erroneous diagnosis of a psychotic disorder. The characteristic symptoms of this seizure disorder are different from those of psychosis in a number of ways, however. They differ, for example, in the rate of onset and the duration of the episode. A number of differences between epileptic seizure phenomena and psychoses are summarized in Table 5-4.

Conversely, there are emotional disorders associated with behaviors that mimic epilepsy. The behaviors are considered hysterical conversion reactions and are called pseudoepileptic seizures. They are typically manifested by voluntary body movements that mimic tonic-clonic seizures. The psychiatric disorders most commonly associated with pseudoepileptic seizures are depression and personality disorders. The differential diagnosis between psychiatric disorder and epileptic seizure disorder is based on clinical observation, the results of laboratory tests, and response to medication. A number of characteristics that distinguish tonic-clonic (grand mal) and pseudoepileptic seizures are summarized in Table 5-5.

### *Interictal Behavioral Alterations and "Epileptic Personality"*

The existence of permanent changes in the behavior of individuals with seizure disorders is a controversial area of research. The controversy focuses on: (1) whether such changes actually exist; (2) if they do exist, the reason for them; and (3) the association of specific types of behavioral alterations with specific seizure disorders.

Research has generally indicated that from 10 to 80 percent of adults with seizure disorders suffer behavioral alterations. The prevalence of change appears to vary with the type of seizure disorder. Specifically, those with simple partial seizures evidence the least change, while those with complex partial seizures evidence the highest rate of interictal behavioral change.

Changes in behavior of individuals with seizure disorders have been variously attributed to: (1) the nature of the underlying dysfunction (e.g., frontal lobe disturbance), (2) the side effects of anticonvulsant medication, (3) personal and social reactions to the seizure disorder, and (4) the existence and location of the epileptic focus.

The existence of an "epileptic personality" is a much debated concept. Research in the area tends to focus on the association of complex partial seizures with personality patterns. Some have asserted that individuals with complex partial seizures experience the greatest degree of interictal behavioral alteration and share recognizable personality characteristics (e.g., religiosity, an interest in the abstract). Other researchers disagree.

Distinctive behavioral patterns have also been attributed to children who have seizure disorders. During infancy and early childhood, motor restlessness and aggressiveness have been noted. During latency years, cognitive deficits and problems around peer relationships have been described. Reactive disorders, such as depression or marked dependence on parents, have been noted in adolescence.

### *Intellectual Functioning*

Functions such as memory skills have been found to deteriorate in individuals with partial and generalized seizures. The loss has been variously attributed to the side effects of anticonvulsant medication, the repeated loss of large numbers of neurons during seizures, and an underlying progressive illness. Depending on its cause, intellectual deterioration may be reversible. For example, memory functions that are impaired as a side effect of an anticonvulsant may return to normal when the drug regimen is changed.

## INFANCY AND CHILDHOOD SEIZURE DISORDERS

As in the case of epileptic seizure disorders, infancy and childhood seizure disorders are the result of paroxysmal alterations in neuronal activity in the brain during which the neuronal discharges become abnormal and uncontrolled. The two disorders encountered most frequently by a psychologist are (1) neonatal seizures and (2) febrile seizures.

### *Neonatal Seizures*

Neonatal seizures may be focal or generalized. Focal seizures are manifested by such behaviors as repetitive blinking, mouth movement, and apnea. The behavioral manifestations are usually subtle. Neonatal seizures often occur within the first week of life. They are the most common neonatal neurological emergency.

### *Febrile Seizures*

Febrile seizures are usually generalized and of short duration. They occur soon after the onset of a fever or at the peak of a fever. When febrile seizures are associated with febrile illness that does not directly effect the CNS (e.g., respiratory illness), they are called benign febrile seizures. Benign febrile seizures are rarely associated with later development of epileptic seizure disorders, learning disorders, or mental retardation. Children with febrile seizure disorders that are associated with febrile illness that does affect the CNS or with pre-existing CNS disturbance, have a less positive prognosis.

Febrile seizures usually occur in children who are between six months and five years of age. They rarely occur in older children who have no earlier history of febrile seizures. Females are less susceptible to febrile seizures than males.

## Etiology of Seizure Disorders

The etiology of seizure disorders falls into three main categories: (1) symptomatic, (2) idiopathic, and (3) genetic.

Symptomatic seizures are those that are symptoms of a diagnosed condition. They may be the consequence of a metabolic abnormality or focal pathology of the central nervous system. For example, an acute systemic metabolic disorder such as hypoglycemia or a drug reaction may trigger epileptic seizures. Epileptic seizures may also be secondary to a bacterial or viral infection. A brain hemorrhage, a contusion, or a tumor may cause seizures due to increased intracranial pressure or metabolic changes in the surrounding neurons. Partial, febrile, and neonatal seizures are typically included in this category.

Idiopathic seizures are those for which there is no detectable cause. This category includes the majority of epileptic seizure disorders in children. Undetected metabolic or structural abnormalities are thought to be involved.

A number of seizure disorders have genetic etiology. Petit mal and febrile seizures are the commonest of this type. Although the specific etiology of tonic-clonic (grand mal) seizures is unknown, they often show a familial pattern of occurrence, suggesting a genetic etiology.

## Diagnosis of Epileptic and Childhood Seizure Disorders

Seizure disorders are not typically associated with clear neurological abnormalities that can be identified in a standard neurological examination. The diagnosis of a seizure disorder is therefore based on the integration of data obtained from: (1) a precise description of the presenting episode(s); (2) the developmental, medical, and family histories; (3) the findings of general medical examination and neurological ex-

**TABLE 5-6. SIDE EFFECTS OF THE COMMONLY PRESCRIBED ANTICONVULSANTS**

| TRADE NAME | GENERIC NAME | COMMON SIDE EFFECTS |
|---|---|---|
| Dilantin | Phenytoin | Nystagmus, ataxia, lethargy |
| Luminal | Phenobarbital | Lethargy, intellectual dulling |
| Mysoline | Primidone | Lethargy, intellectual dulling |
| Tegretol | Carbamazepine | Nystagmus, ataxia, lethargy, nausea, dizziness, rash, blood cell abnormalities |
| Zarotin | Ethosuximide | Nausea, euphoria, headache, drowsiness, blood cell abnormalities |
| Depakene | Valproic acid | Tremor, sedation, gastrointestinal disturbance, liver dysfunction |

amination; and (4) the results of laboratory studies. The choice of laboratory studies will be based on the questions that the neurologist raises in response to the information gathered through the histories and the examinations. Tests for metabolic disorders or infection may be included. The most frequently used medical test for a neurological disorder is an electroencephalogram (EEG). The EEG records the alternating excitation and inhibition of electrical activity of the neurons in the brain, thus revealing electrophysiological dysfunction.

## Treatment of Epileptic and Childhood Seizure Disorders

Attempts are made to control seizures by the use of anticonvulsant medication. Drug therapy is, in fact, the treatment used in the vast majority of cases.

The various disorders have been found to respond differentially to different anticonvulsant medications. Among the most commonly prescribed anticonvulsants are: Dilantin (phenytoin), Luminal (phenobarbital), and Tegretol (carbamazepine). The potential side effects of the anticonvulsants include drowsiness, dizziness, and changes in appetite. Side effects of the commonly prescribed anticonvulsants are summarized in Table 5-6.

## Role of the Psychologist

As noted, the diagnosis and treatment of a seizure disorder is the responsibility of the neurologist. Often, however, it is the psychologist who first raises the question of a possible seizure disorder. Although adults commonly come to the psychologist describing symptoms or expressing concerns about possible seizure phenomena, children do not. Therefore, in order to evaluate a child for an epileptic seizure disorder, the psychologist must rely on his ability to obtain pertinent information. This requires the knowledge of what to look for and what to ask both parent (or guardian) and child.

The psychologist bases the decision to refer a child to a neurologist on a review of: (1) the present condition and presenting problem(s); (2) the developmental, medical, and family histories; (3) the clinical interview; (4) the child's test performance, appearance, and behavior during the course of the evaluation. The information is obtained from: 1) parent (guardian) interview, (2) school report, and (3) clinical observation.

### *Parent (Guardian) Interview*

It is unlikely that a child will be brought first to a psychologist if the parent (or guardian) suspects a seizure disorder; a child is more apt to be brought to a medical doctor. Nevertheless, through careful initial questioning of the parent (or guardian) regarding the presenting condition and problem(s), information suggesting a possible seizure disorder is often obtained. For example, the psychologist may learn that a child complains of stomach pains that start and stop suddenly; or he may hear descriptions of a child "staring into space," even when being spoken to. Both descriptions suggest a seizure disorder and the need for referral to a neurologist for evaluation. Inquiries are made regarding the frequency and duration of such episodes, changes in the nature of the episodes, possible precipitating causes, and alleviating or aggravating factors.

Precise developmental and medical histories are central to the diagnostic process in general, and they may offer the first suggestion of a seizure disorder. Since some seizure disorders have a genetic component, the family history with respect to seizure disorders is obtained (see Appendix 2).

### *School Report*

This report may provide information suggesting a seizure disorder (see Appendix 3).

### *Clinical Observation*

The child is also interviewed about his experiences. The questions are designed to elicit information about the possibility of seizure phenomena. For example, he is asked about hallucinatory experiences and body sensations. If his answers suggest that he might be experiencing seizures, further questions about the frequency and duration of the episodes are asked. Inquiries about the precipitating factors are made (see Appendix 4).

Test performance is scrutinized for possible signs of seizure episodes. For example, skipping squares on the WISC-R Coding subtest, typically interpreted as a sign of distractibility, might also be due to momentary breaks in consciousness.

During the course of the diagnostic evaluation, the psychologist is constantly scanning a child's appearance and behavior for signs of possible seizure phenomena. For example, he notes failures to respond to the environment, automatisms, or jerking movements.

If a seizure disorder is suspected, the psychologist refers a child to a neurologist for a medical evaluation.

**TABLE 5-7. TYPES OF HEADACHES**

I. Intermittent and recurrent headache
   A. Migraine headache
      1. Typical
      2. Common
      3. Classic
   B. Extracranial headache
   C. Cluster Headache
II. Continuous headache
III. Acute headache

Note that the diagnostic evaluation of a child during a seizure does not provide a valid assessment of his intellectual functioning and cognitive skills or his emotional well-being. The quantitative measurements and qualitative assessments made by the psychologist must be validated through reexamination once the seizures are controlled.

## HEADACHES

Headaches are often among the presenting problems of a child referred for an evaluation. While the vast majority of children who complain of headaches do not suffer from a serious neurological condition or disease, headaches are symptoms that cannot be overlooked. First, they are important indications of a child's physical and emotional health. Second, they can impact profoundly on a child's day-to-day activities. Third, they can affect both school performance and social development.

In this section we present an introduction to headaches. We define the types of headaches, summarize their causes, present an overview of diagnostic procedures and treatments used, and describe the role of the psychologist in the diagnostic process.

### Types of Headaches

Headache is defined as pain in the region of the head. There are three major classes of headaches, defined by their clinical presentation: (1) intermittent and recurrent headaches, (2) continuous headaches, and (3) acute headaches. The types of headaches are summarized in Table 5-7 and discussed below.

#### *Intermittent and Recurrent Headaches*

The vast majority of headaches are intermittent and recurrent. They fall into three classes: (1) migraines, (2) extracranial headaches, and (3) cluster headaches. Migraines and extracranial headaches are the types most commonly encountered in the child population. These two classes are briefly described below.

**MIGRAINE HEADACHES.** There are a number of types of migraines. The three most frequently occurring are: (1) the typical migraine, (2) the common migraine, and (3) the classic migraine. Although differing in specific features, all migraines involve severe pain and gastrointestinal disturbance. Hypersensitivity to light is common, as is hypersensitivity to noise. In some instances, migraines are preceded by an aura (e.g., flashing lights). The pain in migraines begins on one side of the head and often becomes bilateral. It is characterized by throbbing.

**EXTRACRANIAL HEADACHES.** Extracranial headaches may cause pain on one or both sides of the head. The pain can range from mild to severe and is usually not characterized by throbbing. There is usually no gastrointestinal upset.

### *Continuous and Acute Headaches*

Continuous headaches are headaches that are continuous and increasingly severe. Acute headaches are suddenly occurring headaches that are characterized by severe and generalized pain.

## Etiology of Headaches

Migraine attacks are thought to be caused by cerebral vascular imbalance. A short period of constriction of the cranial arteries is followed by prolonged dilatation, which leads to increased intracranial pressure. The characteristic throbbing pain of migraine headaches is a reflection of the pulse.

Extracranial headaches in children are often due to damaged or infected tissue in the ears, nose or mouth, or to the contraction of muscles of the neck, scalp, and face. These muscles may contract due to prolonged stress or anxiety. Headaches that are caused by such muscle contraction may be called psychogenic or tension headaches. Children between the ages of six and twelve years who have headaches, usually have this type.

Continuous and acute headaches may be symptoms of serious illnesses or conditions. Possible causes of a continuous headache are: (1) an intracranial mass lesion, such as a tumor or a subdural hemotoma, and (2) an intracranial infection, such as encephalitis, meningitis, or an abcess. Acute headaches may be due to such conditions as hemorrhage or an infection.

## Diagnosis of Headaches

Diagnosis of the type of headache is the province of the medical doctor. The diagnosis is based on the integration of data from: (1) developmental, medical, and family histories; (2) a clinical interview; (3) a physical examination; and (4) laboratory tests and diagnostic imaging tests that might be performed in order to rule out neurological dysfunction and disease states.

## Treatment of Headaches

The first step in the treatment of headaches is diagnosis. Once a diagnosis is made, treatment is started. Treatment of headaches is the professional responsibility of a medical doctor. Assuming a child does not have a serious illness or condition that requires immediate specialized medical intervention, headaches can often be treated effectively by the use of medications. Occasionally other treatment modalities (e.g., feedback therapy) are utilized.

## Role of the Psychologist

A child who complains of headaches is typically treated successfully at home with mild analgesics and rest. The psychologist refers a child to a medical doctor for headache complaints based on a review of: (1) the present condition and presenting problem(s); (2) the developmental, medical, and family histories; and (3) the clinical interview. The information is obtained from: (1) parent (guardian) interview, (2) school report, and (3) clinical observation.

### *Parent (Guardian) Interview*

If the parent (or guardian) does not spontaneously report it, he is asked if his child suffers from headaches. If a child has headaches, a description of a typical headache is obtained, as well as the frequency and duration of the episodes. The character, intensity, and localization of the headaches are ascertained. It is important to inquire about possible precipitating factors, as well as any that exacerbate or relieve the pain. The presence of associated symptoms (e.g., vomiting) is important information.

The history of any headache complaint includes the age of onset. If the character of the headaches has changed, the psychologist notes when these changes occurred.

Familial patterns in the occurrence of headaches have been noted. For that reason, information about the history of headaches in near relatives is requested and may suggest a hereditary disorder (See Appendix 2).

### *School Report*

This report may provide information suggesting headaches (see Appendix 2).

### *Clinical Observation*

A child who complains of headaches should be asked about the symptom. As much information as possible is obtained from the child and the child's description is compared to that of the adult informant.

Depending upon the age of a child, it may be difficult for him to describe the quality, duration, and localization of the headache. In this case, accounts of his behavior during the episode may be the best way to assess the headache (see Appendix 4).

A referral is made to a medical doctor for an evaluation when: (1) previously effective means of treating the headaches no longer work, (2) the character of the headaches has changed, or (3) the headaches interfere with a child's normal daily activities.

## REVIEW QUESTIONS

1. Epileptic seizure disorders occur in approximately 5 percent of all children. True or False?
2. What is epilepsy?
3. Most seizure disorders in childhood are associated with abnormalities discernible on a routine neurological evaluation. True or False?
4. What is an EEG?
5. The two main categories of epileptic seizure disorders are focal and generalized. True or False?
6. A focal seizure never spreads to involve the entire cortex. True or False?
7. Psychomotor seizures are typically manifested by directed violent behavior. True or False?
8. Petit mal and tonic-clonic seizure disorders are the most frequently seen forms of epileptic seizure disorder in children. True or False?
9. All epileptic seizure disorders are inherited. True or False?
10. A psychologist does not diagnose a seizure disorder. True or False?
11. A psychological evaluation of a child who is actively seizing is a valid assessment of the child's intellectual and cognitive skills and emotional well-being. True or False?
12. Headaches in children always indicate a serious neurological condition. True or False?
13. Psychogenic headaches are also called tension headaches. True or False?
14. What are some features of migraine headaches?
15. When should a child be referred to a medical doctor for headache complaints?

# 6

# MEMORY DISORDERS

The majority of children who are referred to a psychologist for an evaluation have learning difficulties. These difficulties are analyzed through the use of a well-designed and comprehensive test battery. Because of the central role of memory throughout the learning process, assessment of memory functions is always a crucial component of a comprehensive psychological evaluation.

In this chapter we present an overview of memory. We summarize the historical background of the study of memory; define memory processes and systems; summarize the neuroanatomical basis of memory; discuss the most dramatic type of memory defect, amnesia; highlight the memory disorders commonly found in children; and present the diagnostic techniques used by the psychologist in examining memory functions.

## HISTORICAL BACKGROUND

Questions about the nature of memory have intrigued philosophers and scientists for over a hundred years. In the eighteenth century, memory was a focal interest of the great philosophers of the day, who were concerned about the different types of memory and the structure of memory.

At the end of the eighteenth century, the first report of an experimental investigation of human memory appeared in the literature. This investigation used a series of nonsense syllables and measured retention of the series after various delay periods. The results, which have been replicated many times since, established that, in long-term memory, duration of the study period and duration of the delay period are important determinants of the amount of information that is recalled (and forgotten).

Investigations of memory during the twentieth century have focused on many

FUNDAMENTALS OF CLINICAL CHILD NEUROPSYCHOLOGY


ISBN 0-8089-1910-5

aspects of long-term memory (e.g., interfering factors) as well as on short-term memory and the overall memory process. The search for the biological basis of memory began in the mid-twentieth century. It was hypothesized that *engrams* (defined as circuits in the brain) are the memory traces. The search for such engrams, however, was fruitless. More recently, as the result of the rapid advances in neurobiology, the biology of memory has been understood in terms of cell membrane alteration and biochemical events. Concurrently, behavioral studies have established that the memory process involves at least three systems: sensory buffer, short-term memory, and long-term memory. The many features of each system are still in the process of being defined.

## MEMORY PROCESSES

One way in which memory phenomena can be conceptualized is by a formulation known as stage theory. According to this theory, there are three stages in every act of remembering: (1) the acquisition of information, (2) the retention of information, and (3) the retrieval of information.

During the acquisition stage, an individual is exposed to an experience that effects a change in the nervous system. This change is commonly referred to as a memory trace. The memory trace, or memory engram, cannot be discerned by available biochemical, neuroanatomical, or radiological techniques. It is most often thought of as a subtle alteration in the structural or biochemical properties of neuronal tissue, or both.

The retention stage occupies the interval between the acquisition and the retrieval of information. Factors inherent in the stimuli (e.g., the frequency of exposure) and others characteristic of the individual (e.g., motivation, cognitive state) interact to determine whether or not a memory trace survives (is retained).

Retrieval is the process of activating a relevant memory trace. An item may be retrieved by: (1) recall or (2) recognition. In recall, an individual spontaneously reconstitutes a previously encountered stimulus. In recognition, an individual responds to a previously encountered stimulus as familiar. For example, fill-in questions on an examination require recall; multiple-choice questions rely upon recognition.

## MEMORY SYSTEMS

Memory involves three CNS functions: (1) the sensory buffer, (2) the short-term memory (STM) system, and (3) the long-term memory (LTM) system.

### The Sensory Buffer

When a stimulus registers on the senses, a sensory image is formed in the sensory

| S | G | Y |
|---|---|---|
| D | M | H |
| Q | X | R |

**Figure 6–1.** Sample of stimulus pattern used in partial report procedure.

buffer, also called the sensory register or sensory information storage (SIS). The sensory buffer is modality-specific. A visual stimulus creates a vivid mental picture, or icon. The sensory register for an auditory stimulus is called an echo.

The sensory buffer holds the experience for a brief period of time after the stimulus is withdrawn. An icon decays in less than one second. An echoic store fades in less than four seconds.

Although it retains information for only a short time, the sensory buffer has substantial storage capacity. This is demonstrated through the partial report procedure. In this experimental procedure, as used for the visual modality, a subject reports only the stimulus in a designated area of the full array of a set of visual stimuli. The critical area is designated after the array is withdrawn, in order to ensure that a subject is using his memory to respond. Figure 6-1 illustrates the type of stimulus pattern used in these studies.

The information held in the sensory buffer is not analyzed. It is "raw material," essentially an exact copy of what was experienced. The purpose of the sensory buffer is to maintain information until higher order analysis assigns the information to an established category.

Forgetting occurs in the sensory buffer when (1) neural firing is stopped by neural adaptation to the input and (2) subsequent input "erases" previous input.

## The Short-Term Memory System

Short-term memory, also referred to as immediate memory, holds a limited number of items for immediate retrieval. The limit of the average adult's short-term memory storage capacity for unrelated items, independent of the mode of presentation, is approximately seven items plus or minus two (Miller's magic number). Items stored in the short-term memory remain available for recall for approximately thirty seconds.

In contrast to the sensory buffer in which items are stored "raw," the short-term memory system stores data that is processed to some degree. For example, there are two short-term memory stores: (1) auditory-verbal and (2) visual. Items are stored in the auditory-verbal memory in acoustical form, even when the material is presented through a different modality, e.g., visually. It is presumed that an individual labels the stimuli, thus recoding the visual data into an acoustical symbol. Maintenance rehearsal, or continually reinserting an item into short-term memory store, also aids short-term memory. An example of maintenance rehearsal is an individual's constant repeating of a telephone number he is about to dial.

Failure in short-term memory is thought to be due to a combination of: (1) trace decay, in which forgetting occurs because the memory trace fades, presumably as a result of a metabolic process and (2) interference, in which items are pushed out of short-term memory by new items entering the system.

## The Long-Term Memory System

Long-term memory retains information for extended periods of time. The capacity of the long-term memory system is enormous.

### *Varieties of Long-Term Memory*

Long-term memory can be subdivided on the basis of: (1) content and (2) the time span between acquisition and retrieval of the information. The content of memory is of two types: (1) generic and (2) episodic.

Generic memory is an individual's memory for items of general knowledge. For example, the answer to the question "Who discovered America?" is an item in generic long-term memory. Generic memory represents the sum total of all that an individual has learned.

Episodic memory is an individual's memory for events in his own life, e.g., what happened yesterday in school.

Long-term memory is subdivided on the basis of time span between information acquisition and retrieval into: (1) recent memory and (2) remote memory. Recent memory refers to the memory for items stored minutes to months ago. Remote memory refers to the memory for items stored in the more distant past.

### *Long-Term Memory Processes*

Information is thought to be transferred from short-term memory to long-term memory for long-term storage. The processes by which this occurs are not clearly understood. It is known that they are affected by features of the information (e.g., relevance) and by characteristics of the individual learner (e.g., the way he rehearses and reorganizes material he is trying to memorize).

Through active rehearsal, an individual apparently reorganizes information. Information may be recoded into larger units (chunks). The recoding may be in the form of: (1) grammatical units or (2) semantic categories. Thus, although the memory for unrelated words is quite limited, an individual may be able to recall large quantities of verbal information if it is organized in sentence form. Similarly, if unrelated items are reorganized into categories, the number of items that can be recalled increases appreciably. Based on critical features, the item may be filed into object categories.

Acoustical representations of the experience are also created and filed, as is information on how to reproduce it.

The retention phase, which entails the consolidation of the memory trace, occurs over a period of time ranging from a few seconds to a few months after the stimulus first registers on the senses. During the early stages of consolidation, the stored information is very vulnerable to alterations in brain processes. Such alterations typically occur as a result of brain insults. If an insult to the brain (e.g., a seizure) occurs within thirty minutes of the formation of a memory trace, the trace is usually lost.

When information is retrieved from long-term memory, it is based on a reconstruction of the associations and representations of the original experience. It is not a duplicate of the original experience. The retrieval of information from long-term storage is generally preceded by an active internal process called a memory search. The success of a memory search is dependent on the accessibility of the memory trace. Access to a memory trace, in turn, may be fostered by a retrieval cue.

Mnemonics are techniques that aid in the retrieval process. Mnemonics facilitate the active reorganization of information to be remembered. Mnemonic methods use verbal reorganization (e.g., use of a rhythm to maintain a series in sequence) and visual imagery (e.g., the method of loci, in which the items to be remembered are envisioned in specific locations, and each location is mentally examined to recall the items).

### *Forgetting*

No one theory of forgetting appears to account adequately for all instances of memory failure. Some of the explanations that have been advanced are:

1. Decay of the memory trace. Forgetting occurs because the memory trace fades over time, as the result of natural metabolic processes.
2. Interference. Forgotten information is not "lost"; rather, its retrieval is interfered with. Interference can occur in two ways:
   a. Retroactive inhibition, in which new learning interferes with remembering of previously acquired information
   b. Proactive inhibition, in which previously learned information interferes with retrieval of new information
3. Change in retrieval cues. The inability to remember information may be due to a difference between cues used at the time of learning and those available at the time of recall.

## Interaction of the Memory Systems

Although presented in isolation, the memory systems interact in complex ways. Information does not simply flow from the sensory buffer to the short-term register to the long-term memory store. Rather, the flow between memory systems is two-directional, may overlap in time, and may not be sequential. For example, items in the short-term memory system are maintained and processed in terms of their relevance,

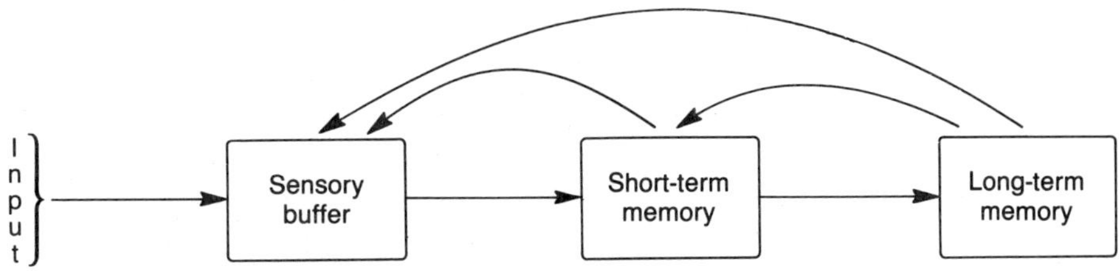


**Figure 6–2.** Interaction among the memory systems.

based on information stored in the long-term memory system. Figure 6-2 is a schematic representation of the interaction among the memory systems.

## NEUROANATOMICAL BASIS OF MEMORY

Memory is mediated by the interaction of cortical and subcortical areas. The subcortical focus of memory is the limbic system, notably the hippocampus. A limbic circuit originates in the hippocampal formation and includes the mammillary bodies and areas of the thalamus. The hippocampi receive most of their information from the temporal lobes, which in turn receive information from the cortical association areas, especially the parietal and frontal regions. (Figure 6-3 illustrates the major structures of the limbic system.)

The sensory buffer and short-term memory have been associated with reverberation within the hippocampal circuit. The sensory buffer has, in addition, been associated with activity of the peripheral (receptive organ) pathways and cortical projection regions.

If there is dysfunction at any point in the limbic circuit, long-term memory is affected. Hemispheric specialization has also been suggested: dysfunction in the hippocampi and thalamus of the dominant hemisphere selectively disrupts verbal learning; dysfunction in the nondominant side disrupts nonverbal learning. It is thought that remote memories are stored in appropriate association regions of the cerebral cortex. As a consequence, these memories are not totally dependent on the limbic system for storage and retrieval and are highly resistant to insults to the brain. Remote memories are lost only when there is dysfunction in the specific association areas themselves.

## AMNESIA

Amnesia is a general term for a severe memory defect that affects long-term

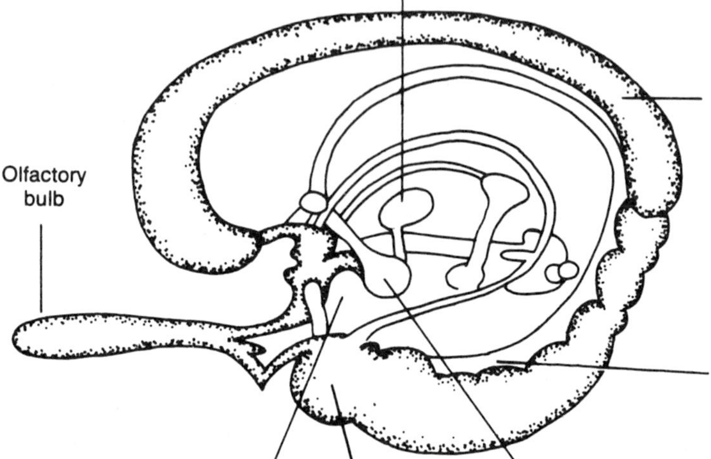


**Figure 6–3.** Major structures of the limbic system. (Adapted with permission from *Clinical Neuropsychology*, 2/e, by K. Heilman and E. Valenstein. Oxford University Press, 1985.)

memory but does not affect short-term memory or general intellectual level. There are two types of amnesias: (1) retrograde and (2) anterograde.

## Retrograde Amnesia

An individual with retrograde amnesia is unable to retrieve memories of experiences that occurred prior to the insult. When faced with a question he cannot answer, he may confabulate (i.e., "fill in" with a memory of an event that occurred earlier). The closer the memory is to the time of the brain insult, the more difficult it is to retrieve. The amnesia is most severe immediately upon regaining consciousness. Although it tends to recede over time, some individuals suffer permanent memory loss.

The underlying mechanism of retrograde amnesia is not clear. The amnesia is thought to be due to interference with the consolidation of the memory trace during the early stage of storage. Thus memories are not shifted from the short-term memory system to the long-term memory system and are forgotten. The amnesia also appears temporarily to interfere with the retrieval process. This interference is reversible, however, and there is typically a regaining of memories over time.

### Anterograde Amnesia

Although able to maintain previous learning, an individual suffering from anterograde amnesia is unable to learn new material. Information can be maintained in short-term memory, as long as it is being rehearsed. There is, however, no transfer from the short-term memory to the long-term memory store. An individual with anterograde amnesia presents as disorganized and confused, since his inability to learn prevents him from accommodating to changes in his environment. He may confabulate in an attempt to fill in memory gaps.

Anterograde amnesia may be transient if the condition causing it is transient; for example, brain swelling due to trauma. The amnesia will be permanent for experiences that occurred during the time of the illness, however. Permanent anterograde amnesia is a characteristic of patients with alcoholic Korsakoff disease.

The mechanism underlying anterograde amnesia is not clear. Current research suggests that anterograde amnesia may be a defect either in the storage of new material in long-term memory or in its retrieval.

## MEMORY DISORDERS IN CHILDREN

Memory disorders in children occur frequently. They, however, often are not recognized. The memory defect is likely to be modality-specific (e.g., auditory or visual), a function of the specific type of memory task (e.g., sequential or spatial), or a function of the nature of the material involved (e.g., nonsense or meaningful). Auditory memory deficits involve sequential information. Visual memory deficits involve sequential or spatial material.

## ASSESSMENT OF MEMORY FUNCTIONS

Assessment of memory functions requires the integration of quantitative and qualitative information. Quantitative assessment is based on a child's performance on standardized tests of memory functions. Qualitative information is obtained from different sources (e.g., reports from parent (or guardian) and school). Representative quantitative and qualitative measures of memory functions are presented in Appendix 6.

### Quantitative Assessment

There are a number of standardized tests of short-term auditory memory. These are typically subtests of tests designed to evaluate complex and multifaceted skills, such as language functions. Standardized tests are also available to assess short-term visual sequential and visual spatial memory functions and recent visual memory. Standardized tests of intelligence and achievement assess a child's generic long-term memory.

Poor performance on a memory test may not be due to a memory problem per se; rather it may be secondary to another problem, such as poor perceptual, graphomotor, or language functions. These functions are assessed to determine their relationship to a child's ability to perform memory tasks. The roles of personality factors are also considered.

### Qualitative Assessment

The qualitative information used to assess a child's memory functions includes data obtained from the following.

**Parent (Guardian) Interview.** Assessment of memory functions begins when the psychologist elicits from the parent (or guardian) information about the child's ability to carry out verbal directions or ease of learning number facts and words for spelling tests.

A medical history, which includes information about serious illnesses and major accidents, is also obtained (see Appendix 2).

**School Report.** A school report is requested and reviewed for the teacher's comments on the child's ability to perform memory-based tasks, e.g., learning the number facts (see Appendix 3).

**Clinical Observation.** Qualitative information about a child's memory functions is obtained from: (1) observing the quality of the child's performance on standardized tests of memory skills, (2) noting the quality of the child's performance on age-appropriate informal tests of memory, and (3) observing the child's spontaneous verbalizations and behavior. One notes the relative ease of performance and the use or the development of memory "tricks" during the course of a test. Attitudes and behavior that interfere with a child's performance are noted; for example, a lack of motivation to do well on the presented task may be apparent (see Appendix 4).

## REVIEW QUESTIONS

1. Memory functions play a peripheral role in learning. True or False?
2. What are the three stages involved in remembering?
3. What is a memory trace?
4. Features of the material to be remembered affect whether or not a memory enters long-term storage. True or False?
5. In what two ways are memories retrieved? Give an example of each.
6. What are the three CNS functions involved in memory?
7. The sensory register holds information for an extended period of time. True or False?
8. What are the limits of short-term memory in terms of time and number of items held?

9. What is the difference between rehearsal in short-term memory and rehearsal in long-term memory?
10. In what ways are items recoded in long-term memory?
11. There is no interaction between the memory systems. True or False?
12. What is amnesia?
13. Memory disorders in children are uncommon. True or False?
14. Memory functions are assessed in a comprehensive psychological evaluation. True or False?
15. Poor performance on a memory test may be secondary to a language disorder. True or False?

# 7

# SENSORY AND PERCEPTUAL DISORDERS

All information about the external environment and the internal state of the body is obtained through the sensory systems. Six sensory systems have been described: (1) visual, (2) auditory, (3) olfactory, (4) gustatory, (5) somatosensory, and (6) balance. Although all of these affect a child's development, the visual, auditory, and somatosensory systems play a central role. The visual and auditory systems provide information about the appearance and sounds of surrounding space. The somatosensory system informs us about sensations arising in the skin such as feelings of pain, touch, and temperature. It also informs us about sensations that originate inside the body, thereby providing information about the state of the musculoskeletal system and the visceral organs.

Even a subtle dysfunction in one of these sensory systems is likely to have a profound effect on a child's development. For example, dysfunction in the auditory system may compromise a child's ability to discriminate speech sounds. As a result, he may have serious difficulty comprehending spoken language and learning to speak. Thus, the evaluation of any childhood learning, behavioral, or emotional disturbance must include an examination of sensory systems to rule out subtle sensory dysfunctions.

This chapter presents an overview of the visual, auditory, and somatosensory systems. We summarize the neuroanatomical basis of these senses; define the major sensory disorders commonly seen by psychologists, especially those seen in children; and discuss their causes and their diagnosis. Sensory disorders that are rarely encountered but that have special value in explicating the functional organization of a particular sensory system are also discussed. The visual system is presented first, followed by the auditory and somatosensory systems.

FUNDAMENTALS OF CLINICAL CHILD NEUROPSYCHOLOGY

ISBN 0-8089-1910-5

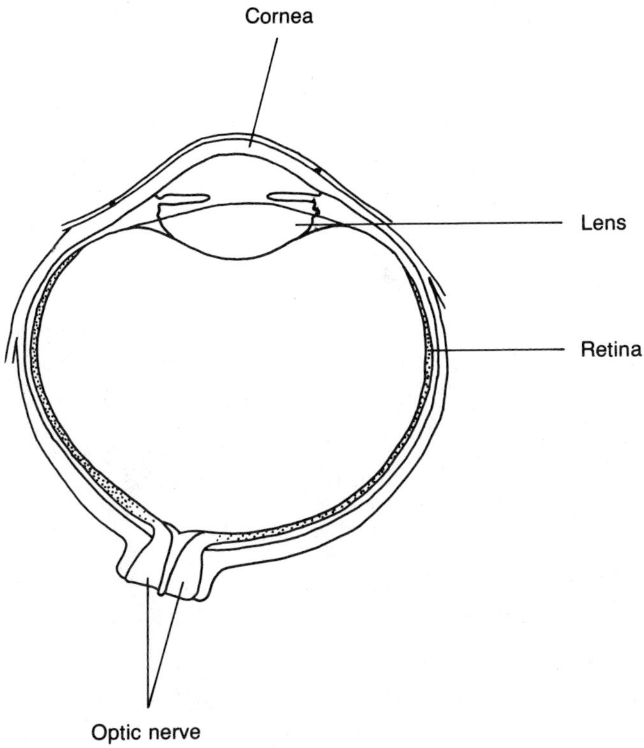


**Figure 7–1.** Major structures of the eye.

## VISUAL SYSTEM

### Neuroanatomical Basis of Vision

The visual image enters the eye through the cornea and lens and is received by the receptors of the visual system. These are the rods and cones. They are located within the retina at the back of each eye. The retina is divided into two areas, which differ functionally and structurally. These are the peripheral and central areas. The peripheral portion of the retina is responsible for peripheral vision and scotopic vision (the ability to see light, dark, and motion). The central portion of the retina is responsible for detailed visual perception and for color vision. The peripheral portion is made up primarily of rods. The central portion is made up predominantly of cones. A simplified diagram of the eye is shown in Figure 7-1.

The visual receptors (rods and cones) in each eye give rise to an optic nerve. The right and left optic nerves converge at the base of the brain to form the optic chiasma. Some fibers go on from there to terminate in the superior colliculus, which is located

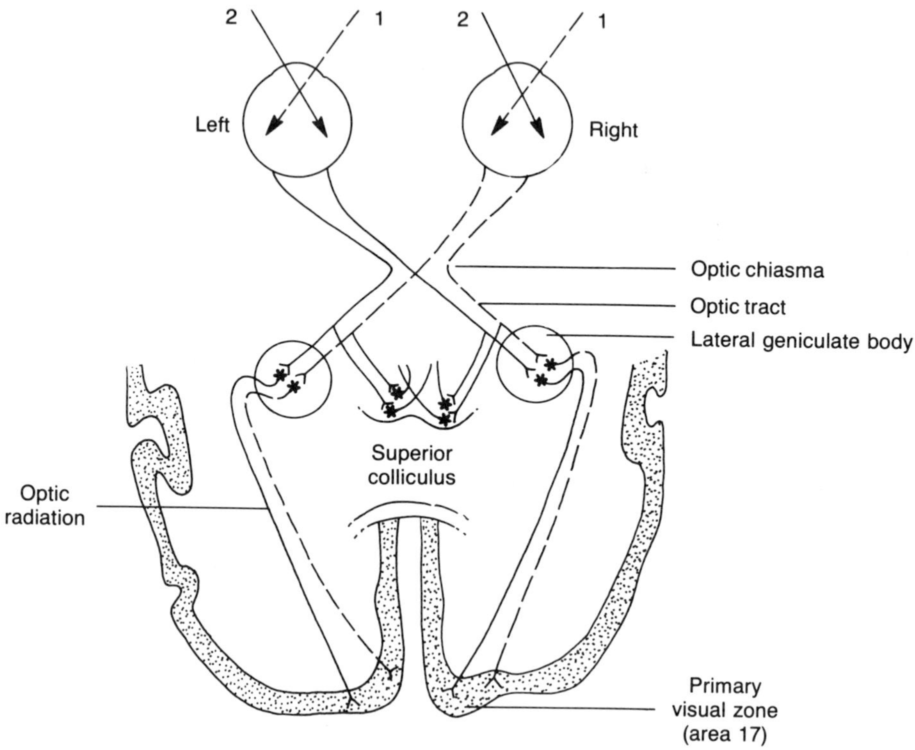


**Figure 7–2.** The visual pathways. (From: *Fundamentals of Neurology* by E. Gardener, copyright © 1964 by W.B. Saunders Co. Reprinted by permission of Holt, Rhinehart, & Winston, Inc.)

in the midbrain. Most fibers, however, proceed from the optic chiasma to form the right and left optic tracts. These tracts ascend first to a major subcortical relay station, the thalamus. Fibers that originate on the right side of the retina proceed to the right lateral geniculate body of the thalamus. Those that originate on the left side of the retina ascend to the left lateral geniculate body of the thalamus. The lateral geniculate nucleus serves as a relay station that sends visual information not only to the cortex but also to reflex centers that control eye movement. From the thalamus, the optic radiation emerges and traverses the temporal lobe. It terminates in the occipital lobe, where the primary visual recepton area of the cortex is located (see Figure 7-2).

## Disorders of the Visual System

Disorders of the visual system can be divided into four groups: (1) disorders of

**TABLE 7-1. DISORDERS OF THE VISUAL SYSTEM**

I. Visual acuity disorders
  A. Myopia
  B. Hyperopia
  C. Blindness
II. Ocular motility disorders
  A. Involuntary or reflexive
    1. Nystagmus
    2. Strabismus
  B. Voluntary
    1. Ocular dysmetria
    2. Ocular dyspraxia
III. Visual field defects
IV. Visual information processing disorders
  A. Visual perceptual and visual recognition
    1. Visual discrimination disorder
    2. Visual agnosia
      a. Simultanagnosia
      b. Object agnosia
      c. Prosopagnosia
      d. Color agnosia
  B. Visual-spatial
    1. Unilateral visual neglect
    2. Topographical orientation defect
  C. Visual constructive
    1. Assembly disorder
    2. Graphomotor disorder

visual acuity, (2) disorders of eye movement, (3) visual field defects, and (4) disorders of visual information processing. They are summarized in Table 7-1 and are discussed below.

Developmental visual disorders in children are likely to resemble those seen in adults. Consistent with the general differences between brain dysfunction in adults and children, however, they tend to be more subtle.

### *Disorders of Visual Acuity*

Visual acuity refers to the ability to detect a visual stimulus accurately. In visual acuity disorders, a child's sensitivity to visual stimuli is disturbed. Visual acuity disturbances range from a subtle degree of nearsightedness (myopia) or farsightedness (hyperopia) to blindness.

### *Disorders of Ocular Motility*

Ocular motility refers to movements of the eyes. It occurs on two levels: (1) involuntary (or reflexive) and (2) voluntary.

Normal binocular vision depends upon involuntary eye movements by means of which both eyes focus on the same object but send slightly different images to the occipital lobe. These disparate images are fused in the occipital lobe. In addition to their role in binocular vision, these eye movements are also crucial to our ability to maintain an unchanged picture of the world as we move around in it. Whenever the position of the body changes, reflexive eye muscle changes are stimulated to move the eyes accordingly. The voluntary control of eye movement permits active exploration of the environment.

Disorders of ocular motility may involve either the involuntary or the voluntary movement of the eyes. These include: (1) nystagmus, (2) strabismus, (3) ocular dysmetria, and (4) ocular dyspraxia.

Nystagmus and strabismus are both disorders of involuntary eye movements. Nystagmus is characterized by involuntary rhythmical or unrhythmical oscillation of one or both eyes. In strabismus, one eye is fixated on a visual target while the other eye is directed elsewhere. Strabismus is commonly called crossed eyes. In both disorders, paired eye movement (also referred to as conjugate eye movement) is affected.

Ocular dysmetria and ocular dyspraxia are disorders of voluntary eye movement. In ocular dysmetria, a child is unable to track a moving target or to look suddenly from one target to another. In ocular dyspraxia, a child is unable to turn his eyes voluntarily in a given direction on command.

### *Visual Field Defects*

In visual field defects a child experiences a loss of vision that may range from a blind spot to loss of half the field of vision (hemianopia).

### *Disorders of Visual Information Processing*

Information processing disorders are the visual disturbances most often seen by the psychologist. Visual information processing entails the analysis, synthesis (integration), and evaluation of visual stimuli. Disorders in the processing of visual information may be clinically manifested in: (1) visual perceptual and visual recognition disorders, (2) visual-spatial disorders, and (3) visual constructive disorders.

#### Visual Perceptual and Visual Recognition Disorders

***Visual Discrimination Disorder.*** The most basic task in processing visual information is that of visual discrimination. Visual discrimination is involved in: (1) the recognition of an embedded figure, (2) the identification of an object on the basis of prominent features, (3) the identification of an object on the basis of partial presentation, and (4) the differentiation of figure and ground in a visual array. A visual discrimination disorder is manifested in a child's failure to perform these tasks.

***Visual Agnosia.*** This is a rare visual disorder in which a child is unable to recognize familiar stimuli that are presented visually despite intact sensory processing, language, and general intelligence. A remarkable feature of visual agnosia is that it is often specific for a particular class of stimuli. Indeed, the disorder is classified in terms of the specific visual simuli that cannot be recognized. We describe four of the visual agnosias. These are: (1) simultanagnosia, (2) object agnosia, (3) prosopagnosia, and (4) color agnosia.

*SIMULTANAGNOSIA.* This term refers to a condition in which a child is unable to recognize or abstract the meaning of a complex visual stimulus (e.g., panorama) despite accurate recognition of its individual parts.

*OBJECT AGNOSIA.* In this condition, a child is unable to recognize a familiar stimulus (e.g., a dog) despite intact visual recognition of its component parts (e.g., tail, legs, ears). He can recognize the object by smell, sound, or touch.

*PROSOPAGNOSIA.* This is the inability to recognize familiar faces. Although able to correctly describe a face and to recognize people by smell, sound of voice, and other cues, an individual with this disorder cannot recognize faces on the basis of visual cues alone.

*COLOR AGNOSIA.* In this disorder, a child is unable to recognize colors. Color matching and memory of the color of familiar items remain intact (e.g., bananas are yellow, grass is green).

**VISUAL-SPATIAL DISORDERS**

***Unilateral Visual Neglect.*** This disorder is manifested by a child's failure to respond to stimuli in one or the other lateral visual fields.

***Topographical Orientation Defect.*** This disorder is manifested by a child's inability to describe spatial characteristics of his environment or to orient himself in space and on a map.

**VISUAL CONSTRUCTIVE DISORDERS.** Children with visual constructive disorders are unable to appreciate the visual-spatial relations among the component parts of a visual whole and as a consequence are unable to put the parts together correctly. Visual constructive disorders may affect the performance of two different types of tasks: (1) assembly (e.g., block design) and (2) graphomotor.

The demands placed on a child's linguistic, visual-spatial, and motor skills are not the same for the two classes of tasks. Thus, it is not uncommon for a child to do poorly on one kind of visual constructive task and do well on another depending on the nature of his underlying dysfunction.

## Causes of Visual Disorders

Visual sensory information passes through the cornea and the lens and is received by the retina. Further processing occurs at each relay station within the visual pathway. Thus, there are a number of sites of possible dysfunction within the visual system. These localized dysfunctions, in turn, cause distinctive visual sensory and perceptual disorders.

Visual information is consistently transmitted contralaterally. Information in the right visual field of each eye is transmitted to the left cerebral hemisphere. The reverse is true for the left visual field.

Unilateral dysfunction in pathways before the level of the optic chiasma causes loss of vision in one eye. Dysfunction of the crossing fibers at the optic chiasma causes loss of vision in the temporal half of each eye. This is manifested by a slight constriction of the visual field, which is frequently unnoticed by a child. Unilateral dysfunc-

**TABLE 7-2 SIGNS OF VISUAL DISTURBANCE BY SITE OF DYSFUNCTION**

| Site | Signs |
|---|---|
| **Cornea and Lens** | Partial to total loss of sensitivity to visual stimuli; Myopia; Hyperopia; Distortion of image |
| **Retina** | Partial to total loss of sensitivity to visual stimuli; Visual field defects |
| **Optic Nerve** | Partial to total loss of sensitivity to visual stimuli; Visual field defects; Unilateral blindness |
| **Optic Chiasma** | Partial to total loss of sensitivity to visual stimuli; Visual field defects; Unilateral blindness |
| **Optic Tract** | Visual field defects |
| **Lateral Geniculate Bodies** | Visual field defects |
| **Optic Radiation** | Visual field defects |
| **Brain Stem** | Nystagmus |
| **Cerebellum** | Nystagmus |
| **Cranial Nerves** | Nystagmus; Strabismus |
| **Cortex** | Ocular dysmetria; Ocular dyspraxia; Visual field defects; Visual discrimination disorders; Visual agnosia; Visual-spatial disorders; Visual constructive disorders; Blindness |

tion in pathways beyond the level of the optic chiasma causes loss of vision of the contralateral (opposite) side of space. When there is unilateral dysfunction of the optic tract, it is associated with loss of the contralateral half of the visual field of each eye. Unilateral cortical dysfunction causes loss of vision of the contralateral half of space. Cortical dysfunction, in addition to affecting the visual field, also affects the perception of complex aspects of visual stimuli. Bilateral cortical dysfunction causes partial or complete cortical blindness.

A broad range of visual disturbances are listed according to site of dysfunction in Table 7-2.

### *Disorders of Visual Acuity*

Disorders of visual acuity are associated with dysfunction of the cornea, lens, or any component of the visual system from the retina to the cortex.

### *Disorders of Ocular Motility*

Involuntary or reflexive eye movements are governed by the cranial nerves. Thus, nystagmus and strabismus are associated with this type of dysfunction. However, nystagmus can also be associated with dysfunction in the vestibular system, the cerebellum, or the brain stem.

Voluntary eye movement is governed by the motor cortex of the frontal lobe. Thus, dysfunction in the motor cortex provides a sufficient explanation for ocular dysmetria. In ocular dyspraxia, dysfunction of the language regions of the dominant hemisphere is also implicated.

### *Visual Field Defects*

Visual field defects are always due to specific lesions in the primary visual pathway. The site and extent of dysfunction determine the pattern of loss of vision. For example:

1. When dysfunction is limited to the outer fibers of an optic nerve, peripheral vision is affected (peripheral field restriction).
2. When only the central portion of the nerve is affected, only central vision is affected. This disorder is referred to as a central scotoma (blind spot).
3. Unilateral dysfunction of the optic tract results in half-field blindness. The inner boundary of the blind spot is irregular unless damage to the tract is total.
4. Bilateral cortical dysfunction results in blindness.

Certain dramatic visual field defects, by site of dysfunction, are illustrated in Figure 7-3.

### *Disorders of Visual Information Processing*

These disturbances always indicate dysfunction in higher cortical centers, as follows.

**VISUAL PERCEPTUAL AND VISUAL RECOGNITION DISORDERS.** Visual discrimination disorders are associated with occipital lobe dysfunction. The visual agnosias are typically associated with bilateral dysfunction variously involving the occipital and parietal lobes.

**VISUAL-SPATIAL DISORDERS.** These disorders are commonly associated with unilateral, usually right-sided, parietal dysfunction.

**VISUAL CONSTRUCTIVE DISORDERS.** These disorders are usually, but not always, associated with bilateral cortical dysfunction.

## Diagnosis of Visual Disorders

Visual disorders cannot be evaluated without clear information on visual acuity. This is obtained through ophthalmological examination.

The psychologist's diagnosis of a visual disorder depends upon both quantitative and qualitative data. Qualitative data are obtained from: a parent (guardian) interview (Appendix 2), a school report (Appendix 3), and clinical observation (Appendix 4). Clinical observation provides information about the quality of a child's performance on: (1) standardized tests that depend upon visual skills, (2) age-appropriate visual tasks, and in (3) spontaneous behavior and verbalizations.

Representative quantitative and qualitative measures of visual disorders are summarized in Appendix 7.

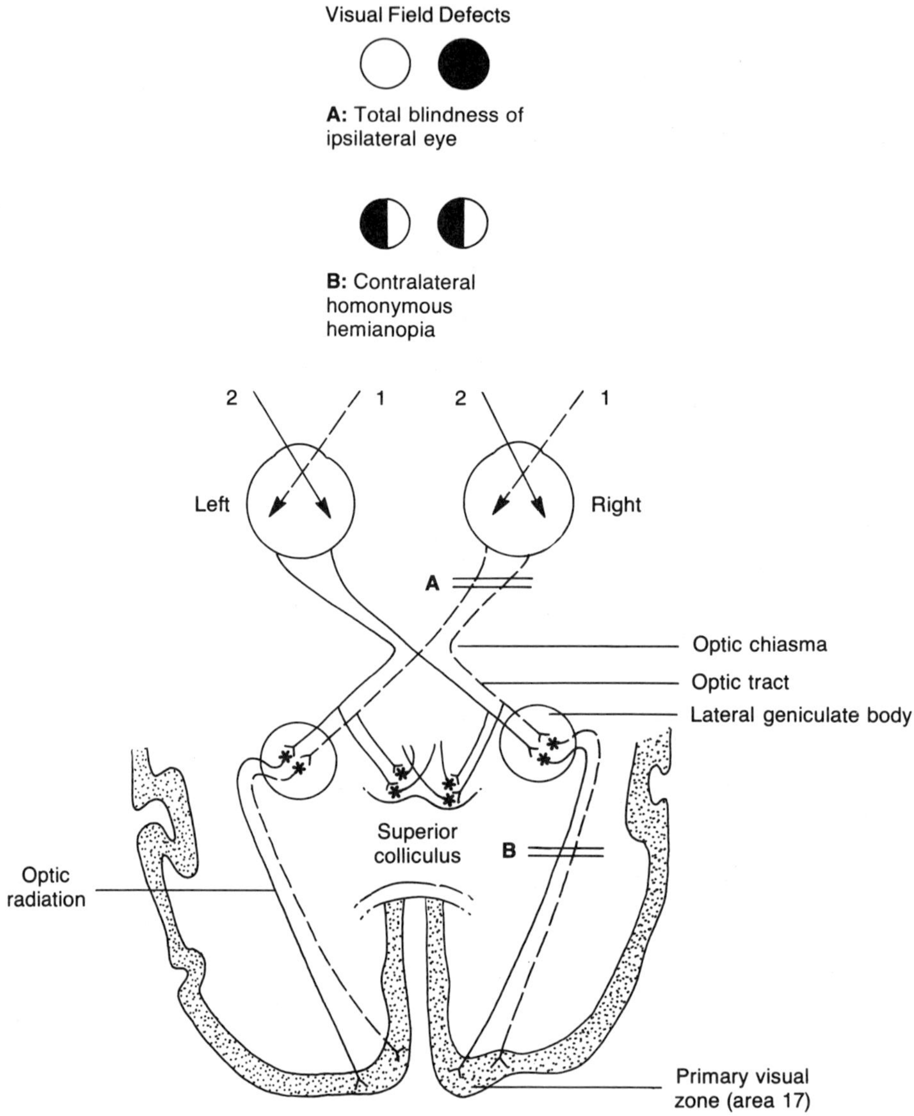


**Figure 7–3.** Representative visual field defects by site of dysfunction in visual pathways: *A*. Total blindness of ipsilateral eye. *B*. Contralateral homonymous hemianopia. (From: *Fundamentals of Neurology* by E. Gardener, copyright © 1964 by W.B. Saunders Co. Reprinted by permission of Holt, Rhinehart, & Winston, Inc.)

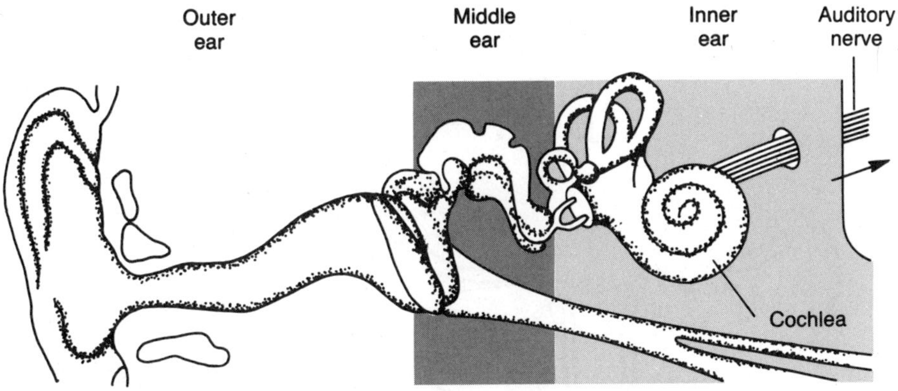


**Figure 7–4.** Major structures of the ear. (From: *Understanding Human Behavior*, 5/E, by J.V. McConnell. Copyright © 1986 by CBS College Publishing. Reprinted by permission of Holt, Rhinehart, & Winston, Inc.)

## AUDITORY SYSTEM

### Neuroanatomical Basis of Hearing

Sounds are transmitted to the brain through the ear. They enter the outer ear, then the middle ear, and finally the inner ear. The auditory receptors are in the cochlea, located in the inner ear. These receptors, known as hair cells, are located within the organ of Corti in the cochlea. The organ of Corti serves as a frequency analyzer. Its organization is tonotopic, with the lowest frequency tones monitored at the apex and the highest frequency tones monitored at the base of the organ. A simplified diagram of the ear is shown in Figure 7-4.

The auditory nerve arises from the cochlea in each ear. The fibers of the auditory nerve ascend first to the superior olivary nucleus in the medulla. At this point, the auditory tract divides. Some fibers continue on an ipsilateral course, while others cross to pathways in the contralateral midbrain region. The two fiber bundles of the auditory tract ascend through the lateral lemniscal pathway. Some fibers branch off from the lateral lemniscal pathway to the cerebellum and to the ascending reticular formation in the brain stem. The main tracts, however, synapse in the inferior colliculus, which is located in the roof of the midbrain. From there, they ascend to the medial geniculate body of the thalamus. Finally, the fiber bundles project to the primary auditory area of the cortex. This is located in Heschl's gyrus in the transverse temporal gyrus, a portion of the superior temporal gyrus. It is located within the medial temporal lobe. A diagram of the auditory pathways is shown in Figure 7-5.

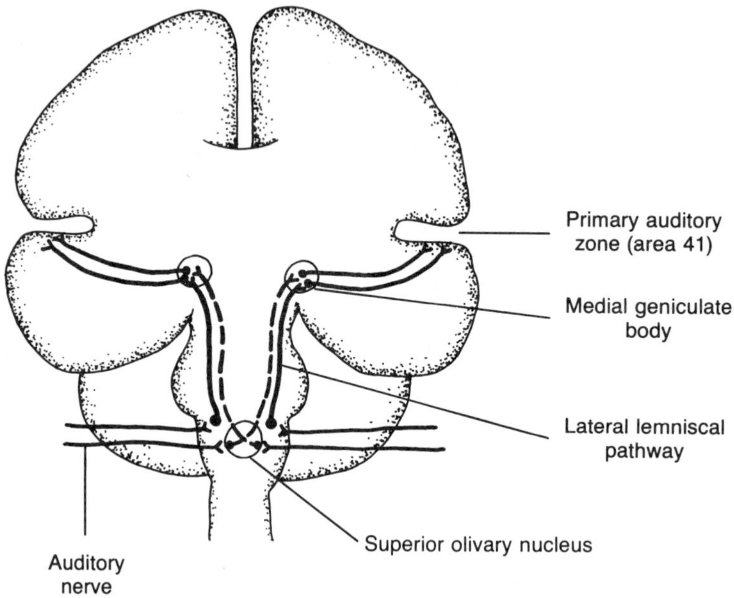


**Figure 7–5.** The auditory pathways. (From: *Fundamentals of Neurology* by E. Gardener, copyright © 1964 by W.B. Saunders Co. Reprinted by permission of Holt, Rhinehart, & Winston, Inc.)

## Disorders of the Auditory System

Auditory system disorders that may be seen by the psychologist are those involving: (1) sensitivity to sounds (deafness), (2) disturbance in the discrimination of sounds, and (3) disturbance in the recognition of sounds (auditory agnosia). These are summarized in Table 7-3 and discussed below.

Developmental auditory disorders in children are likely to resemble those seen in adults. Consistent with the general differences between brain dysfunction in adults and children, however, they tend to be more subtle.

### *Deafness*

Auditory disorders that involve diminished sensitivity to sounds, or deafness, can be divided into two general groups: (1) conductive deafness and (2) nerve deafness.

**CONDUCTIVE (OR TRANSMISSION) DEAFNESS.** A child with conductive deafness usually experiences diminished sensitivity to sounds of all frequencies. If sound vibrations are strong enough or near enough to the head to set bones of the skull in motion, however, bone vibrations may reach the cochlea and be heard. Thus, a child with a conductive disturbance, who is typically unable to hear ordinary face-to-face

**TABLE 7-3. DISORDERS OF THE AUDITORY SYSTEM**

I. Deafness
   A. Conductive (or transmission) deafness
   B. Nerve deafness
      1. Diminished sensitivity to sounds
      2. Difficulty discriminating speech
II. Auditory discrimination disorder
III. Auditory agnosia
   A. Total auditory agnosia
   B. Verbal auditory agnosia (word deafness)

conversations, may be able to process the same conversations when they take place via the telephone.

**NERVE DEAFNESS.** Nerve deafness is defined by the particular aspect of auditory processing that is affected: (1) sensitivity to sounds or (2) ability to discriminate speech.

The first category, loss or diminution of sensitivity to sounds, may involve sounds only within a limited frequency range or within a wide frequency range. In the second category, for example, a child has difficulty discriminating spoken language. In a mild case, the disturbance might be apparent only when a conversation is taking place in a crowded and noisy room. In a severe case, it might be apparent even in a quiet environment.

### *Auditory Discrimination Disorder*

An auditory discrimination disorder is characterized by an inability to discriminate sounds. In fairly mild cases, it may involve only sounds (either nonspeech or speech) that are very much alike. In severe cases, it involves inability to discriminate any speech or nonspeech sounds.

### *Auditory Agnosia*

Auditory agnosia, a very rare disorder, is characterized by inability to recognize familiar sounds despite normal hearing. This disorder may involve nonspeech or speech sounds.

**TOTAL AUDITORY AGNOSIA.** This involves a disturbance in the ability to recognize nonspeech and speech sounds.

**VERBAL AUDITORY AGNOSIA (WORD DEAFNESS).** This involves an inability to recognize speech sounds, with preserved ability to recognize nonspeech sounds (and to process language that is visually presented).

## Causes of Auditory Disorders

Auditory information is transmitted via the ear and auditory receptors to the auditory nervous system pathways. Auditory input is bilateral, each ear transmitting

**TABLE 7-4. SIGNS OF AUDITORY DISTURBANCE BY SITE OF DYSFUNCTION**

| |
|---|
| **OUTER AND MIDDLE EAR** |
| Conductive (transmission) deafness |
| **COCHLEA** |
| Nerve deafness |
| **AUDITORY NERVE** |
| Nerve deafness |
| **SUBCORTICAL STRUCTURES** |
| Nerve deafness |
| Partial to total loss of ability to localize sounds |
| Partial to total loss of ability to integrate sounds received by the two ears |
| **CORTEX** |
| Partial to total loss of ability to discriminate complex speech sounds |
| Partial to total loss of ability to discriminate complex rhythmic combinations of nonspeech sounds |
| Partial to total loss of ability to discriminate sounds that are simultaneously presented to both ears |
| Auditory agnosia |

information to both sides of the brain. The majority of nerve fibers, however, cross to the auditory cortex opposite the receiving ear. Dysfunction at different sites results in distinct patterns of auditory loss.

Dysfunction of the outer and middle ear, the cochlea, and the auditory nerve disturbs a child's sensitivity to sounds. Dysfunction of the auditory nerve may also affect discrimination of speech.

Dysfunction of subcortical auditory pathways results in disturbed ability to localize sounds in space. It also results in disturbed ability to discriminate speech sounds that are embedded in noise and to integrate the sounds received by the two ears.

Cortical dysfunction is reflected in deficient ability to discriminate the more subtle, complex, frequency combinations found in certain speech sounds and complex rhythmic combinations found in music. These disturbances reflect dysfunction in the left and right auditory cortex, respectively.

Unilateral lesions in the auditory cortex also result in impaired discrimination of complex sounds received by the contralateral ear. Such lesions may, in addition, interfere with the ability to discriminate sound stimuli that are simultaneously presented to both ears.

Bilateral lesions of the auditory cortex seriously interfere with ability to discriminate complex sounds but do not appreciably alter the ability to detect sound.

Signs of auditory system disturbance by site of dysfunction are summarized in Table 7-4.

### *Deafness*

**CONDUCTIVE (OR TRANSMISSION) DEAFNESS.** This disorder is caused by dysfunction of the outer or middle ear.

**NERVE DEAFNESS.** Nerve deafness, which involves loss of sensitivity to sounds, is associated with dysfunction of the peripheral auditory pathway; namely, the cochlea. Dysfunction of the cochlea typically affects a restricted frequency range, most often the high range. Total unilateral destruction of the cochlear nerve results in deafness on that side.

Nerve deafness that involves deterioration of the ability to discriminate speech sounds, is associated with dysfunction of the auditory nerve or auditory brain stem pathway. A unilateral defect within the central auditory pathway does not cause total deafness on that side, because each ear transmits information to the brain bilaterally.

#### *Auditory Discrimination Disorder*

An auditory discrimination disturbance may be the result of dysfunction of the cochlea, the auditory nerve, the subcortical structures, or the cortex.

#### *Auditory Agnosia*

**TOTAL AUDITORY AGNOSIA.** Total auditory agnosia is a result of bilateral dysfunction of the temporal lobe.

**VERBAL AUDITORY AGNOSIA (WORD DEAFNESS).** Verbal auditory agnosia has been associated with left-hemisphere and bilateral disturbance of the temporal lobe.

### Diagnosis of Auditory Disorders

Auditory disorders cannot be evaluated without clear information on auditory acuity. This is obtained through a comprehensive audiological evaluation.

The psychologist uses both quantitative and qualitative data to diagnose auditory disorders. Qualitative assessment is based on: a parent (guardian) interview (Appendix 2), a school report (Appendix 3), and clinical observation (Appendix 4). Clinical observation provides information about the child's performance on: (1) standardized tests, (2) age-appropriate tasks, and in (3) spontaneous behavior and verbalizations.

In the course of the evaluation, the psychologist takes note of: (1) inadequate responsiveness to sounds and (2) inappropriate responses to verbal communication.

Representative quantitative and qualitative measures of auditory disorders are summarized in Appendix 8.

## SOMATOSENSORY SYSTEM

The somatosensory system transmits and processes stimulus information originating both outside and inside the body. This information can be divided into several categories: (1) light touch, (2) pressure touch, (3) kinesthetic, (4) temperature, and (5) pain.

Because the tactile somatosensory system is the one of most concern to the psychologist, we focus on it here. We also discuss body schema and its disorders.

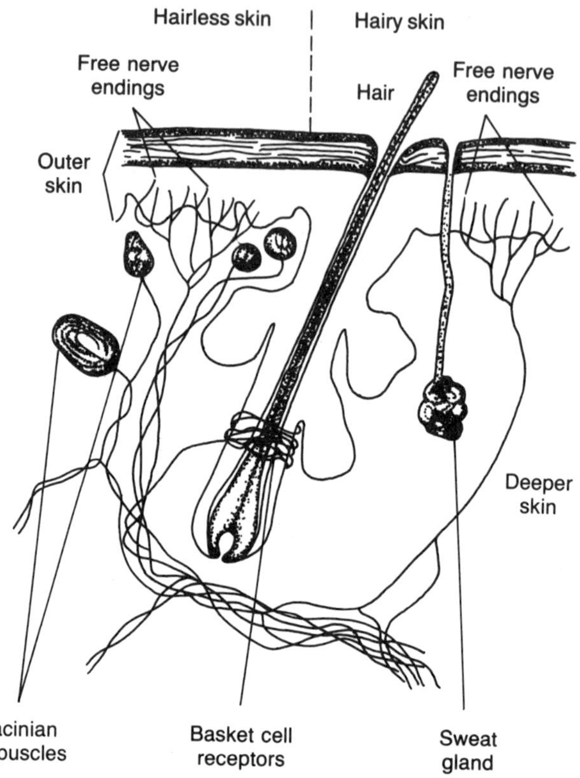


**Figure 7–6.** Major structures of the skin. (From: *Understanding Human Behavior*, 5/E, by J.V. McConnell. Copyright © 1986 by CBS College Publishing. Reprinted by permission of Holt, Rinehart, & Winston, Inc.)

While not explicitly a function of the somatosensory system, body schema is more closely akin to it than to other areas discussed in the book. Both touch and body schema disorders have important effects upon a child's cognitive and emotional development. For example: an infant's and a young child's early learning relies heavily upon tactile sensations, which arise through his active exploration of the environment. Certain pre-academic and academic skills, such as counting on the fingers and the development of automatic left-right work patterns, also depend upon both tactile sensations and body schema. An adequate self-concept depends, in part, upon an intact body schema. And so on.

## Neuroanatomical Basis of Touch

The tactile senses have several different types of receptors. These include: (1) basket cell receptors, (2) pacinian corpuscles, and (3) free nerve endings. They are differentially distributed in hairy and hairless skin and in outer and deeper skin layers. A schematic diagram of the skin is shown in Figure 7-6.

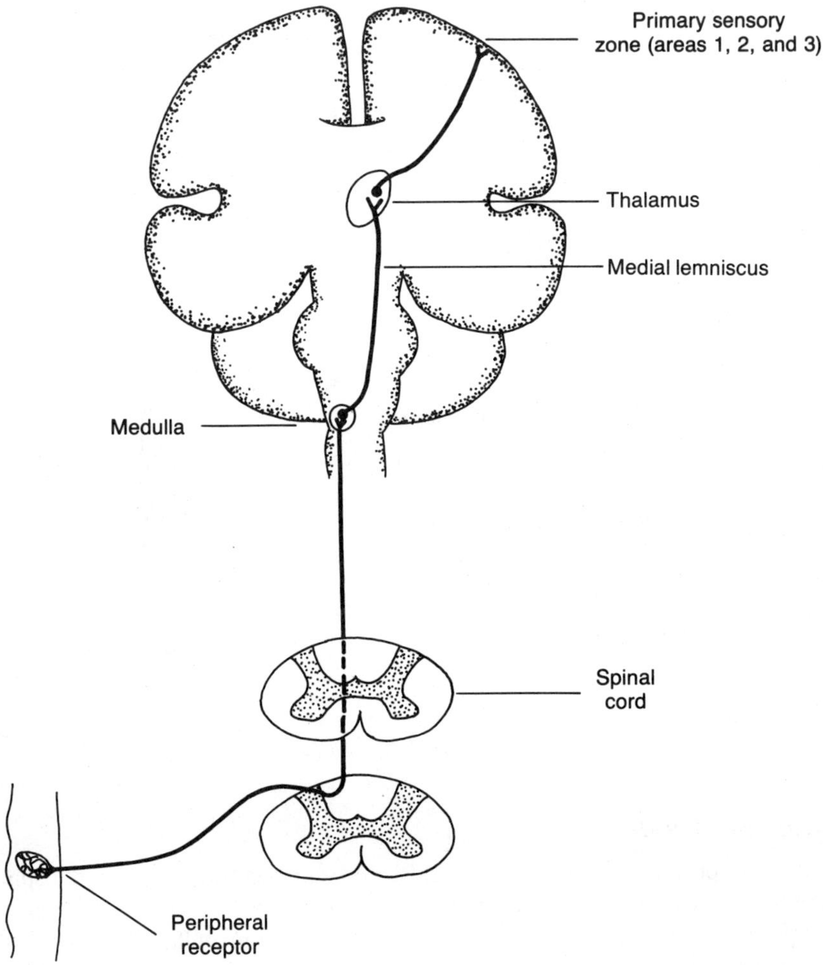


**Figure 7–7.** The lemniscal pathways. (From: *Fundamentals of Neurology* by E. Gardener, copyright © 1964 by W.B. Saunders Co. Reprinted by permission of Holt, Rinehart, & Winston, Inc.)

There are two central nervous system pathways which process tactile information. These are: (1) the lemniscal system and (2) the spinothalamic system. The lemniscal system is involved in the transmission of information regarding light touch and pressure stimuli. The spinothalamic system is involved in the sensations of diffuse touch as well as those of pain and temperature. Since the psychologist is most likely to encounter disturbances of light touch and pressure stimuli, we focus only upon the lemniscal system.

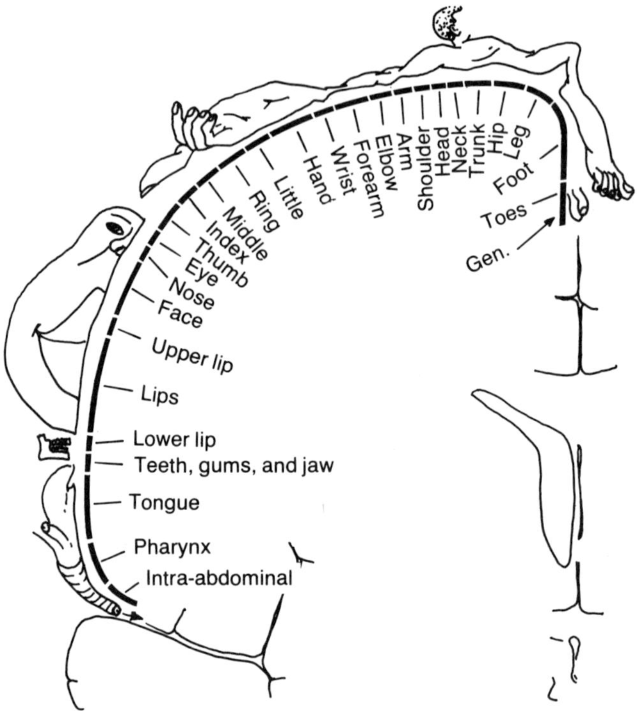


**Figure 7–8.** Sensory homunculus. (Reprinted with permission of Macmillan Publishing Company from *The Cerebral Cortex of Man* by W. Penfield and T. Rasmussen. Copyright © 1950 by Macmillan Publishing Company, renewed by T. Rasmussen.)

### *Lemniscal System*

The peripheral receptors of the lemniscal system send messages to the spinal cord. This information is then transmitted through the nerve fibers of the ipsilateral lemniscal pathway within the spinal cord. At the level of the medulla, all the impulses cross to the opposite side and ascend to the thalamus via a tract called the medial lemniscus. From here, the axons project to the corresponding lemniscal somatosensory area of the cerebral cortex located in the postcentral gyrus of the parietal lobe. (See Figure 7-7.) Areas of the body with the highest receptor density have the largest representation in this cortical region. This representation is not a function of body-part size but rather of the degree of tactile sensitivity that a body region requires. For example, the mouth has greater representation in the cortex than the back. The schematic representation of the body in the parietal cortex is called the sensory homunculus. Figure 7-8 depicts the sensory homunculus.

## Disorders of Touch

There is a broad range of touch disorders and they vary in the complexity of the

**TABLE 7-5. DISORDERS OF THE TACTILE SOMATOSENSORY SYSTEM**

| |
|---|
| I. Tactile localization disorder |
| II. Two-point discrimination disorder |
| III. Double simultaneous discrimination disorder |
| IV. Agraphesthesia |
| V. Haptic imperception |
| VI. Astereognosis |

sensory processing involved. For example, some involve merely the detection of a tactile stimulus and others involve the recognition of an object through manipulation. We describe six disorders: (1) tactile localization, (2) two-point discrimination, (3) double simultaneous discrimination, (4) agraphesthesia, (5) haptic imperception, and (6) astereognosis. The disorders are summarized in Table 7-5 and discussed below.

Touch disorders in children mimic those seen in adults. However, they tend, once again, to be more subtle.

**TACTILE LOCALIZATION DISORDER.** This disorder is characterized by inability to localize a stimulus on the skin.

**TWO-POINT DISCRIMINATION DISORDER.** This disorder is characterized by inability to discriminate between the sensations arising from a single touch stimulus and those arising from two simultaneous nearby touch stimuli.

**DOUBLE SIMULTANEOUS DISCRIMINATION DISORDER.** In this disorder, a child is unable to appreciate the sensations arising from one of two stimuli simultaneously applied to the skin on corresponding body sides.

**AGRAPHESTHESIA.** This disorder is characterized by inability to recognize a shape, number, or letter that is "written" on the hand.

**HAPTIC IMPERCEPTION.** This disorder is characterized by inability to recognize the shape, size, or texture of an object touching the skin.

**ASTEREOGNOSIS.** In this disorder, a child is unable to recognize an object on the basis of its three-dimensionality through palpation.

## Causes of Touch Disorders

Somatosensory processing takes place at the receptor level and also at relay stations within the central somatosensory pathways. Receptor or peripheral nerve dysfunction and spinal cord dysfunction result in the partial to total loss of sensitivity to touch. Subcortical dysfunction within the central pathway results in deficient ability to detect touch. Cortical dysfunction, by contrast, results in impairment of tactile detection and of complex tactile perception. Unilateral cortical lesions impair complex touch perception on the contralateral side of the body. They also result in a lateralized diminution of the ability to detect tactile stimulation. When there is a very large unilateral lesion in the somatosensory receiving area of the parietal cortex, a serious loss of tactile detection on the opposite body side follows.

All six touch disorders previously described are the result of dysfunction in the cortex. Specifically, they are the result of dysfunction of the postcentral gyrus of the parietal

**TABLE 7-6. SIGNS OF TOUCH DISTURBANCE BY SITE OF DYSFUNCTION**

| |
|---|
| **RECEPTOR OR PERIPHERAL NERVE** |
| Partial to total loss of sensitivity to touch |
| **SPINAL CORD** |
| Partial to total loss of sensitivity to touch |
| **SUBCORTICAL PATHWAY** |
| Partial to total loss of ability to detect touch |
| **CORTEX** |
| Partial to total loss of ability to detect touch |
| Defect in tactile localization |
| Defect in two-point discrimination |
| Defect in double simultaneous discrimination |
| Agraphesthesia |
| Haptic imperception |
| Astereognosis |

lobe. The dysfunction site is usually contralateral to the affected body part. A unilateral lesion can, however, produce a bilateral disorder. The common signs of tactile disturbance that are associated with lemniscal system dysfunction are listed by site of dysfunction in Table 7-6.

### Diagnosis of Touch Disorders

The psychologist's diagnosis of touch disorders is based upon quantitative and qualitative data. Qualitative data are obtained from a parent (guardian) interview (Appendix 2), a school report (Appendix 3) and clinical observation (Appendix 4). Clinical observation provides information about the quality of a child's performance on: standardized tests that depend upon tactile processes, age-appropriate tasks, and spontaneous behavior and verbalizations. The diagnosis of touch disorders requires referral for a neurological examination.

Appendix 9 summarizes representative quantitative and qualitative measures of touch disorders.

## BODY SCHEMA DISORDERS

Body schema (or image) disorders are disturbances in a child's spatial perception of his own body. A number of body schema disorders may be seen by the psychologist. These include: (1) finger agnosia, (2) right-left disorientation, (3) the Gerstmann syndrome, and (4) neglect disorders, which are the most severe and also the rarest of the body schema disorders. Body schema disorders are outlined in Table 7-7 and discussed below.

### Finger Agnosia

Finger agnosia is characterized by a child's inability to recognize or identify his own and/or someone else's fingers.

**TABLE 7-7. DISORDERS OF BODY SCHEMA**

I. Finger agnosia
II. Right-left disorientation
  A. In reference to self
  B. In reference to environment
III. Gerstmann syndrome
  A. Finger agnosia
  B. Right-left disorientation
  C. Writing disorder (dysgraphia)
  D. Arithmetic disorder (dyscalculia)
IV. Neglect
  A. Tactile extinction
  B. Anosognosia
  C. Dressing apraxia
  D. Denial

**DEVELOPMENT OF FINGER RECOGNITION AND IDENTIFICATION SKILLS.** The ability to recognize and identify fingers depends upon both complex visual-spatial and language skills. These develop gradually during childhood. A six-year-old child, for example, is expected to be able to identify a single finger of his own when it is touched in his view by an examiner. During the next six years, he gradually develops the ability to identify his own fingers when they are hidden from his view and touched by an examiner. At age twelve, he is still not expected to perform at the adult level in a task that involves identifying pairs of fingers hidden from his view and simultaneously touched by an examiner. Only after this ability is in place, probably during the middle teenage years, is he expected to be able to localize fingers on a schematic model (used in place of his own hands).

### *Causes*

Finger agnosia is usually associated with left parietal dysfunction.

### *Diagnosis*

There are quantitative measures of finger agnosia. In order to utilize these tests, the psychologist must establish that a child has:

1. Adequate verbal memory.
2. Adequate ability to apply verbal labels.
3. Age-appropriate conceptual development.

The psychologist also uses qualitative measures in assessing finger agnosia. These qualitative measures involve careful observation of the child's fine motor behavior and evaluation of his developmental history.

## Right-Left Disorientation

Right-left disorientation is characterized by a child's inability to recognize his own right and left body parts and the right and left sides of his environment.

**TABLE 7-8. DEVELOPMENTAL STAGES OF RIGHT-LEFT ORIENTATION**

I. Orientation toward one's own body
  A. Naming single lateral body parts touched by examiner
  B. Pointing to single lateral body parts on verbal command
  C. Executing double uncrossed movements on verbal command (e.g., touching right knee with right hand)
  D. Executing double crossed movements on verbal command (e.g., touching right knee with left hand)

II. Orientation toward one's own body without visual cues
  A. Naming single lateral body parts touched by examiner
  B. Pointing to single lateral body parts on verbal command
  C. Executing double uncrossed movements on verbal command (e.g., touching right knee with right hand)
  D. Executing double crossed movements on verbal command (e.g., touching right knee with left hand)

III. Orientation toward confronting examiner
  A. Naming single lateral body parts
  B. Pointing to single lateral body parts on verbal command
  C. Imitating uncrossed movements of the examiner (e.g., putting right hand on right knee)
  D. Imitating crossed movements of the examiner (e.g., putting right hand on left knee)

IV. Combined orientation toward one's own body and confronting examiner
  A. Placing specified hand on specified part of confronting examiner on verbal command (e.g., pointing to examiner's left hand with right hand)

(Adapted from Heilman and Valenstein, 1985).

**DEVELOPMENT OF RIGHT-LEFT ORIENTATION SKILLS.** A child of six years is expected to be able to identify his own right and left body parts. A child of nine years is expected to be able to cross the midline in following two-part commands (e.g., touch your right hand to your left eye). By the time a child is about twelve years of age, he should be able to identify right and left body parts on a confronting examiner. The stages of right-left orientation development are summarized in Table 7-8.

### *Causes*

Right-left disorientation is generally associated with left or bilateral parietal dysfunction.

### *Diagnosis*

There are quantitative tests of right-left disorientation. By and large, however, qualitative measures are utilized in assessing this disorder. One such measure involves observation of the quality of a child's responses to right-left directions during the examination. Another involves observation of a child's spontaneous behavior and verbalizations and his ability to perform a number of age-appropriate tasks. These tasks are derived directly from the right-left orientation developmental timetable outlined above.

## Gerstmann Syndrome

The existence of the Gerstmann syndrome, a very rare disorder, as a unitary clinical entity is somewhat controversial. As described, it consists of four principal disturbances: (1) finger agnosia, (2) right-left disorientation on self, (3) writing disorder (also referred to as dysgraphia), and (4) arithmetic disorder (also referred to a dyscalculia). In addition, children with the Gerstmann syndrome often have language and constructional disturbances.

### *Causes*

The Gerstmann syndrome is commonly associated with parietal dysfunction.

### *Diagnosis*

Diagnosis of the Gerstmann syndrome depends upon the use of both quantitative and qualitative measures. In the first place, a child's competence in the writing and arithmetic areas is established through quantitative and qualitative measures outlined in Chapters 10 and 11, respectively. The presence of finger agnosia and left-right disorientation is established on the basis of the criteria described above.

## Neglect Disorders

Disorders of neglect, which are extremely rare in children, are characterized by a failure to appreciate one side of the body. This may manifest itself through: (1) tactile extinction, (2) anosognosia, (3) dressing apraxia, and (4) denial.

An individual with a tactile extinction disorder fails to report a tactile stimulus on one hand when both hands are stimulated simultaneously, but can detect a tactile stimulus on that hand when it alone is touched. In anosognosia, an individual denies that one side of his body is paralyzed. Dressing apraxia is characterized by a failure to dress both sides of the body. An individual with a denial disorder does not recognize one side of his body.

### *Causes*

Neglect disorders are commonly associated with right parietal dysfunction.

### *Diagnosis*

The diagnosis of neglect disorders depends upon the careful observation of an individual and evaluation of his history.

## REVIEW QUESTIONS

1. What are the names of the visual receptors and where are they located?
2. Name two disorders of ocular motility.
3. Define a visual field defect.
4. What are the characteristics of visual agnosia?
5. Unilateral cortical dysfunction is usually implicated in visual constructive disorders. True or False?
6. What are the main symptoms of conductive deafness?
7. Verbal auditory agnosia is associated with deafness. True or False?
8. What is haptic imperception?
9. Astereognosis is a visual information processing disorder. True or False?
10. The Gerstmann syndrome is a unitary disorder. True or False?
11. Which brain region is implicated in touch disorders?
12. Which brain region is implicated in word deafness?
13. Right-left disorientation is a part of the Gerstmann syndrome. True or False?
14. What are the three main types of visual processing disorders?
15. Dysfunction of central auditory pathways results in diminished sensitivity to sound. True or False?

# 8

# MOTOR DISORDERS

Motor problems are readily visible. It is wrong to conclude, however, that they are therefore relatively easy to diagnose. Diagnosis of the main motor disturbances that do not reflect higher cortical dysfunction is relatively straightforward; the diagnosis of those motor disturbances that do reflect higher cortical dysfunction is not.

In this chapter we describe the major classes of motor disturbance associated with neurological dysfunction. We first define the neuroanatomical basis of motor function; then describe the motor disorders commonly seen by the psychologist as well as those less frequently or even rarely encountered that serve to illustrate the relation between damage to the motor system and behavior; discuss the causes of these motor disorders; summarize the timetable of motor skill development; and discuss the diagnosis of motor disorders in general.

## NEUROANATOMICAL BASIS OF MOTOR FUNCTIONS

The control of human muscular activity arises from the CNS and the peripheral nervous system.

The CNS controls muscular activity of the trunk and limbs. This is accomplished at a number of different levels within the nervous system. From the lowest to the highest level, control arises from: 1) the spinal cord, 2) the brain stem, 3) the cerebellum, 4) the basal ganglia, and 5) the cortex. Each level provides a different level of control. For example, the spinal cord controls activity of specific muscles and the cortex controls activity that involves large numbers of distinct combinations of different muscles.

The peripheral nervous system controls muscular activity of the head and neck via the cranial nerves. The motor pathways for the cranial nerves ascend from the brain stem to the cortex.

FUNDAMENTALS OF CLINICAL CHILD NEUROPSYCHOLOGY


ISBN 0-8089-1910-5

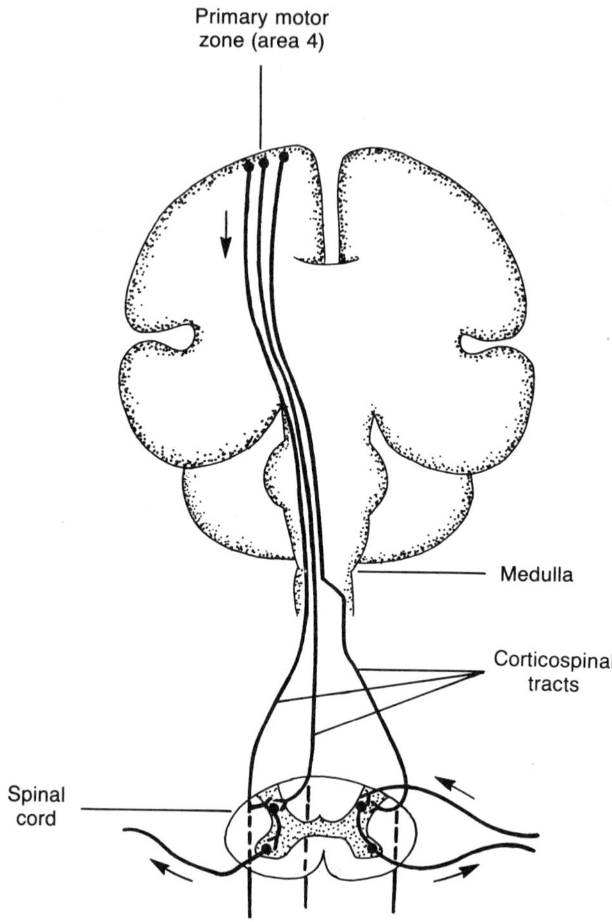


**Figure 8–1.** Corticospinal tracts. (From: *Fundamentals of Neurology* by E. Gardener, copyright © 1964 by W.B. Saunders Co. Reprinted by permission of Holt, Rinehart, & Winston, Inc.)

The functional interaction of two motor systems is central to the control of human motor functions. These are: 1) the pyramidal system and 2) the extrapyramidal system.

## Pyramidal System

The pyramidal system initiates, controls, and maintains voluntary motor activity via a pathway that consists of upper and lower motor neurons. The upper motor neurons of the pyramidal system originate in the motor cortex, which is located in the frontal lobe, and terminate in the spinal cord. Lower motor neurons originate at the level of the brain stem or spinal cord and directly innervate the skeletal muscles. Motor impulses

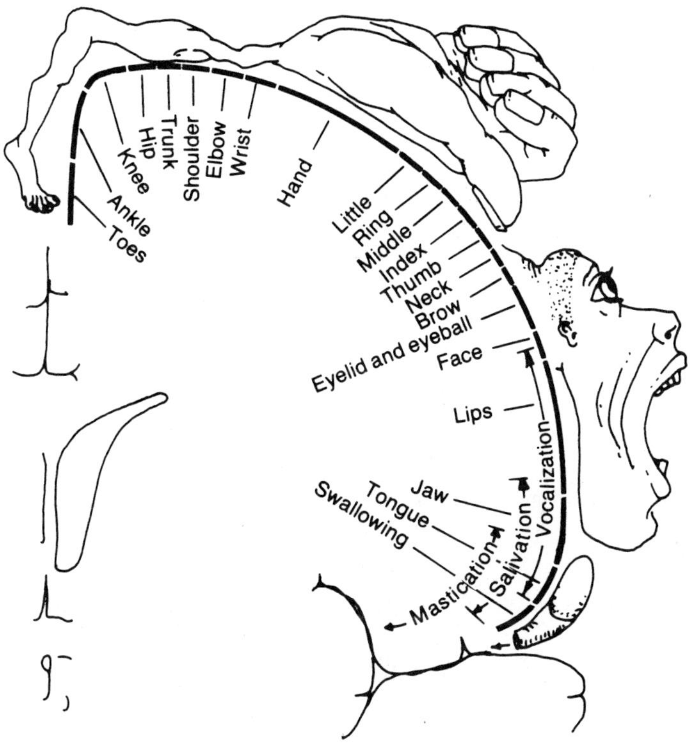


**Figure 8–2.** Motor homunculus.(Reprinted with permission of Macmillan Publishing Company from *The Cerebral Cortex of Man* by W. Penfield and T. Rasmussen. Copyright © 1950 by Macmillan Publishing Company, renewed 1978 by T. Rasmussen.)

originate in the upper motor neurons and descend through the brain, the brain stem, and the spinal cord via fibers in the corticospinal tract. At the level of the medulla in the brain stem, 80 percent of the fibers cross to the other side. This crossing is responsible for the predominantly contralateral motor control of the body by the brain. Some upper motor neurons synapse directly with lower motor neurons in the anterior horns of the lateral columns of the spinal cord. Others make intermediary connections within the corticospinal tract. Nerve fibers from the anterior horns directly innervate the muscles. A simplified diagram of the corticospinal tracts is shown in Figure 8–1.

In the precentral gyrus of the frontal lobes, the head and the body are represented contralaterally and in proportion to the fineness of motor control required of the body part. The motor homunculus depicts the representational pattern (see Figure 8-2).

## Extrapyramidal System

The extrapyramidal system mediates: (1) alterations and adjustments in the body's

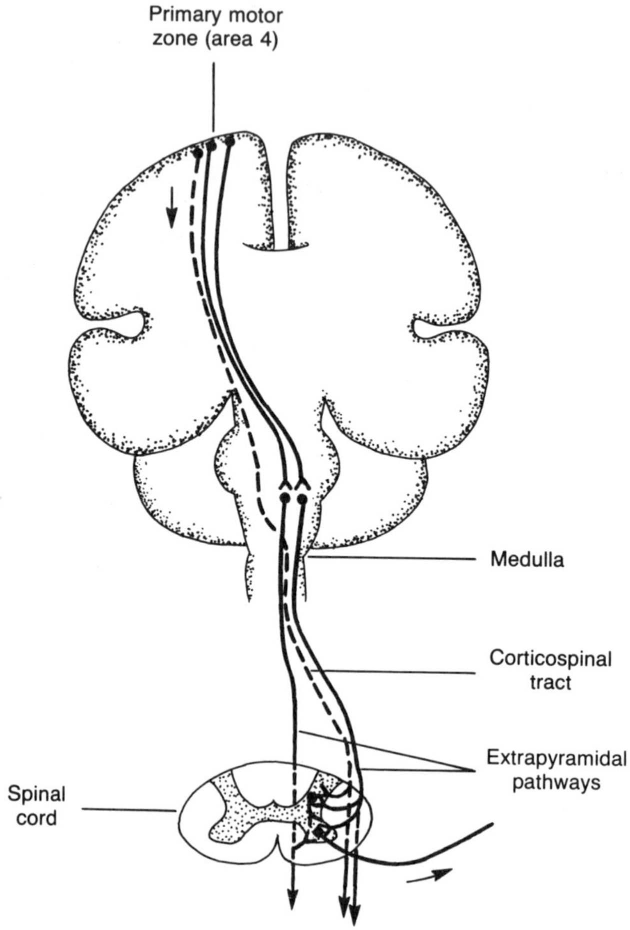


**Figure 8–3.** The extrapyramidal pathways, with corticospinal tract drawn to illustrate relationship between the two motor systems. (From: *Fundamentals of Neurology* by E. Gardener, copyright © 1964 by W.B. Saunders Co. Reprinted by permission of Holt, Rinehart, & Winston, Inc.)

posture and (2) coordination of the movements initiated by the pyramidal system. Like the pyramidal system, the extrapyramidal system utilizes upper and lower motor neurons. The upper motor neurons of the extrapyramidal system originate at the cortical level; the lower motor neurons originate at the level of the brain stem or spinal cord and directly innervate the muscles. The extrapyramidal system encompasses parts of the cerebellum and brain stem and several subcortical structures, including the basal ganglia. A simplified outline of the extrapyramidal pathways is seen in Figure 8–3.

**TABLE 8-1. DISORDERS OF THE MOTOR SYSTEM**

I. Tone disorders
   A. Hypotonia
   B. Hypertonia
II. Strength disorders
   A. Paralysis
   B. Paresis
III. Coordination disorders
   A. Gross motor disturbance
   B. Fine motor disturbance
IV. Abnormal involuntary movements
   A. Tremors
   B. Tics
V. Abnormal associated movements
   A. Mirror movement
VI. Learned skilled motor act disorders
   A. Ideomotor
   B. Ideational
VII. Perseveration

### Interacting Systems

Although the pyramidal and extrapyramidal pathways are themselves remarkably simple, they are affected by a complex set of interacting systems. The initiation of voluntary movement occurs by means of cortical impulses that activate the upper motor neurons. The precise timing and control of movements, once initiated, is accomplished by sensory feedback. Visual receptors, proprioceptors, somatosensory receptors, and the vestibular nuclei in the brain stem are activated by muscle activity, and the resulting sensory impulses are transmitted by complex regulatory pathways to upper motor neurons, whose activity is modified accordingly.

Muscles are rarely, if ever, fully relaxed. At rest, they are maintained at a constant low level of activity by a continual barrage of motor impulses. This constancy is, again, controlled by sensory feedback. Proprioceptors in the muscle sense the state of tension and communicate this via sensory pathways to somatosensory projection areas in the brain that, in turn, signal the upper motor neurons. This constant low level of activity is referred to as muscle tone, and it serves to keep the muscles in an optimal state of readiness.

## MOTOR DISORDERS

The motor consequences of nervous system dysfunction are generally divided into two classes: (1) disorders of muscle tone and strength seen as (a) paralysis or (b) weakness; and (2) disorders of the initiation, control, and maintenance of motor activity. The latter class of motor disorders is seen as: (a) disturbed coordination, (b) abnormal voluntary movements, (c) abnormal associated movements, (d) disturbed performance of learned skilled motor acts, and (e) perseveration. The disorders are summarized in Table 8–1 and discussed below.

Motor disorders in children are likely to resemble those seen in adults. Consistent with the general differences between brain dysfunction in adults and children, motor disorders seen in children tend to be more subtle.

## Disorders of Tone and Strength

Muscle tone is reflected in resistance when an individual's limb is moved passively through the range of motion. There are two classes of muscle tone disorders. These are: (1) hypotonia and (2) hypertonia.

Hypotonia is manifested by reduced resistance. Because normal resistance is slight, hypotonia may be difficult to detect.

Hypertonia is manifested by excessive resistance. There are two types of hypertonia, referred to as rigidity and spasticity. In rigidity, there is excessive resistance throughout the range of movement, independent of the speed of manipulation. In spasticity, there is excessive resistance throughout the range of movement that increases in proportion to the speed of manipulation.

A decrease in muscle strength is often the most prominent sign of motor system dysfunction. Muscle strength disorders may be divided into two groups: (1) paralysis and (2) paresis. Paralysis is defined as a total lack of muscle strength. Paresis refers to a weakness, or partial diminution of muscle strength.

## Disorders of Coordination

A common referral symptom or concern expressed by parents is that a child seems clumsy or poorly coordinated. Because motor coordination is a well-defined function of the central nervous system, the psychologist must always carefully consider possible underlying brain dysfunction as a basis of apparent clumsiness.

Two types of coordination problems are frequently seen by the psychologist. These are: (1) gross motor disturbances and (2) fine motor disturbances. Gross motor disturbances involve movements, such as walking, that are dependent upon the large muscles. Fine motor disturbances involve movement of the fingers. The two types of coordination difficulties may be seen together. More frequently, they are seen in isolation. For example, it is common to see a child who stumbles over his own feet but skillfully manipulates the smallest objects.

## Abnormal Involuntary Movements

There is a large variety of abnormal involuntary movements. Two types commonly seen by the psychologist working with children are: (1) tremors and (2) tics.

Tremors are defined as continual rhythmic shaking of the limbs. All tremors disappear during sleep and are exacerbated by stress and anxiety. Tremors fall into two main categories: (1) postural (also called resting) and (2) intention. Postural tremors

**TABLE 8-2. TIC SYNDROMES OF CHILDREN**

I. Gilles de la Tourette
II. Transient tic of childhood
III. Multiple tic of childhood/adolescence
IV. Invariant tic beginning in childhood

are most prominent during rest and are initially suppressed during intentional movements. As performance of a task progresses, they reemerge. Intention tremors are prominent during movement and become more pronounced during the performance of a task.

Tics are repetitive, stereotyped movements of single and multiple muscle groups. They commonly involve the face and neck but may also involve other body parts. They are often seen as rapid blinking, grimacing, and coughing. They can be temporarily controlled. They are exacerbated by stress and anxiety and diminished by relaxation. They disappear during sleep.

Tics are quite often seen in children. Four types are common: (1) Gilles de la Tourette's syndrome, (2) transient tic of childhood, (3) multiple tic of childhood/adolescence, and (4) invariant tic beginning in childhood (see Table 8-2). Gilles de la Tourette's syndrome is a chronic multiple tic syndrome in which a child develops verbal tics (usually seen as involuntary cursing) as well as multiple motor tics. Typically, the syndrome appears in children between the ages of two and fifteen years and varies in severity over the ensuing years. Transient tic syndromes usually last less than one year, while multiple tic syndromes of childhood and adolescence may last for years, ending in adolescence. Invariant tic syndromes commonly persist throughout an individual's life.

### Abnormal Associated Movements

Normal associated movements include such behavior as the pendular swinging of the arms while walking, spontaneous facial expressions, and the general body movements accompanying coughing, sneezing, and yawning.

The most common type of abnormal associated movement seen in children is called mirror movement. In mirror movement, or overflow, voluntary movements on one side of the body are mirrored on the opposite side of the body. Mirror movement most often involves hand and finger movements.

A tendency toward bilateral mirror movement is normal in preschool children. In a child over the age of nine, the presence of bilateral mirror movement that cannot be suppressed by attention and effort is diagnostically significant. Unilateral mirror movement at any age is considered cause for concern.

### Disorders of Learned Skilled Motor Acts

Motor disorders that involve the inability to initiate or plan learned skilled movements upon verbal command are called apraxias or dyspraxias. The former are acquired disorders. The latter are developmental disorders. We describe only the dyspraxias, as they are the type most often seen in children. There are two general classes of dyspraxia: (1) ideomotor and (2) ideational.

Ideomotor dyspraxia is the type of dyspraxia typically seen in children. It is characterized by an inability to perform accurately (pantomime) on verbal command a previously learned simple motor task that can be performed spontaneously, (e.g., blow a kiss or wave good-bye).

Ideational dyspraxia is a disturbance in the ability to perform accurately (pantomime) upon verbal command a previously learned complex (i.e., multistep or multicomponent) motor task that can be performed spontaneously (such as make a bed). These disorders cannot be accounted for on the basis of motor weakness, sensory loss, or failure to understand the verbal direction.

### Perseveration

Perseveration is characterized by the inappropriate repetition of a particular motor act (e.g., a written or spoken word, a gesture). It is commonly seen in children who have difficulty planning ahead, solving problems, and switching cognitive strategies.

## CAUSES OF MOTOR DISORDERS

Motor disturbance can be a reflection of dysfunction at a large number of sites within the nervous system. Signs of motor disturbances by site of CNS dysfunction are summarized in Table 8–3.

### Disorders of Tone

Hypotonia is associated with dysfunction of the basal ganglia or the cerebellum. Hypertonia is associated with dysfunction of projections into the corticospinal tracts or with dysfunction at the cortical level. Rigidity is associated with basal ganglia dysfunction. Spasticity is associated with cortical dysfunction.

### Disorders of Strength

Dysfunction of the corticospinal tract is associated with paralysis or paresis below the dysfunction site. Usually, when a dysfunction site is in the brain stem or cortex, a hemiparesis results; when it is in the spinal cord, paraparesis or quadriparesis results.

### Disorders of Coordination

Disorders of gross and fine motor coordination are associated with basal ganglia dysfunction and dysfunction of the cerebellar circuits. Disorders of fine motor

**TABLE 8-3. SIGNS OF MOTOR DISTURBANCE BY SITE OF CNS DYSFUNCTION**

| |
|---|
| **SPINAL CORD** |
| Paralysis |
| Paresis |
| **BRAIN STEM** |
| Paralysis |
| Paresis |
| **CEREBELLUM** |
| Hypotonia |
| Paralysis |
| Paresis |
| Gross motor discoordination |
| Fine motor discoordination |
| Intention tremor |
| **BASAL GANGLIA** |
| Hypotonia |
| Rigidity |
| Paralysis |
| Paresis |
| Gross motor discoordination |
| Fine motor discoordination |
| Postural tremors |
| **CORTEX** |
| Spasticity |
| Paralysis |
| Paresis |
| Fine motor discoordination |
| Apraxia/Dyspraxia |
| Perseveration |

coordination may also be associated with dysfunction of the frontal cortex. Because good coordination depends upon normal muscle tone and strength, it also depends upon the nervous system components that govern these functions.

## Abnormal Involuntary Movements

Postural tremors are associated with dysfunction of the controlling functions of the basal ganglia. Intention tremors are associated with cerebellar dysfunction. Tremors can also reflect endogenous chemical changes in the brain or can be a side effect of some classes of medication (e.g., phenothiazines). The latter is a condition called tardive dyskinesia. It is usually irreversible.

Tics may be psychogenic in origin. They may also be the result of diffuse brain dysfunction. Some tics and tic syndromes respond to medications that block dopaminergic receptors in the brain. These may reflect disturbance in specific neurochemical brain pathways.

## Abnormal Associated Movements

Abnormal associated movements are commonly associated with dysfunction in the pyramidal system.

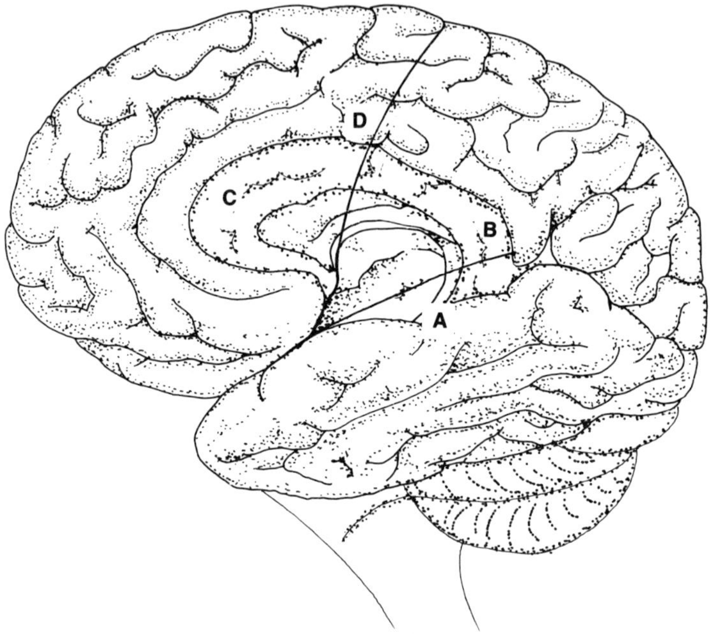


**Figure 8–4.** Regions involved in control of the right hand in performing a skilled motor act on verbal command: *A*. Wernicke's area, mediating comprehension of verbal command: *B*. Association area, mediating integration of verbal command with kinesthetic memories; *C*. Frontal region, mediating evocation of motor memories; *D*. Motor strip, mediating performance of the motor act.

### Disorders of Learned Skilled Motor Acts

These disorders are often associated with a disconnection between the language regions of the dominant hemisphere and the frontal regions concerned with motor programming (Figure 8–4).

### Perseveration

Perseveration is commonly associated with dysfunction of the frontal cortex.

## MOTOR SKILL ACQUISITION TIMETABLE

Motor activity is present during gestation and developmental primacy of the motor system over the sensory systems is well-established during the second trimester.

**TABLE 8-4. HIGHLIGHTS OF MOTOR DEVELOPMENT DURING THE FIRST 15 MONTHS**

| | MOTOR SKILL | | |
|---|---|---|---|
| AGE | SITTING | LOCOMOTOR | MANIPULATION |
| newborn | Flaccid when held to sit, unable to hold head upright | Primitive walking reflex, lying on stomach pulls legs under self | Primitive grasp reflex |
| 1 month | Begins to hold head upright when held in sitting position | | |
| 2 months | | | Reaches for object |
| 3 months | Holds head upright when held in sitting position | | |
| 4 months | | | |
| 5 months | Sits with support, holds back straight | | |
| 6 months | Sits in high chair | | Deliberately grasps object |
| 7 months | Sits alone | | |
| 8 months | | Stands with help | Grasps with thumb and opposite fingers |
| 9 months | Bends forwards when sitting | Stands holding onto furniture, moves by sliding on stomach | Thumb-opposite finger grasp well-developed |
| 10 months | | Crawls | |
| 11 months | | Walks when led | |
| 12 months | | Pulls self to a standing position by holding onto furniture | |
| 13 months | | | |
| 14 months | | Stands alone | |
| 15 months | | Walks alone | |

Development of motor skills is a function of the development of the nervous sytem: the growth of pathways between neurons, increasing myelination of nerve fibers, and the development of specific brain regions. Motor control emerges in a sequential fashion as follows: 1) from central body areas (i.e., upper arms and legs) to outer areas (i.e., fingers and toes), 2) from head to foot, and 3) from large muscles to small muscles.

The newborn's motor behavior consists primarily of primitive reflexes. These are reflexive responses to certain stimuli. For example, the turning of the head toward the touch on a cheek (which is called the rooting reflex). At around four months, primitive reflexes diminish and new reflexes appear. They involve responses to certain body movements. For example, extension of the arms when the body is tilted forward. Though reflexes persist, motor control soon emerges and is seen in the development of sitting, locomotor, and manipulation skills. Basic competence in these areas is apparent by age fifteen months. Continued growth of locomotor and manipulation skills consists of elaboration of the basic motor skills previously acquired. These elaborations (e.g., skipping in the locomotor area, writing in the manipulation area) depend upon the interaction of two crucial factors: (1) continued development of essential nervous system regions and (2) practice.

Highlights of the motor skill acquisition timetable during the first fifteen months of life are presented in Table 8-4.

## DIAGNOSIS OF MOTOR DYSFUNCTION

The assessment of motor functions requires the integration of both quantitative and qualitative information. Quantitative measures are provided by standardized tests. Qualitative information is obtained from many different sources (e.g., reports from parents, special clinical procedures). A summary of representative quantitative and qualitative measures is provided in Appendix 10.

Of the major motor disorders, the one that requires the most refined diagnosis is dyspraxia. Because dyspraxia is a disturbance of learned skilled motor acts that is *not* a reflection of impaired motor function per se, it is always of critical importance to establish the integrity of motor functions before making this diagnosis.

### Quantitative

Of the disorders discussed in this chapter, the psychologist uses standardized tests of gross motor and fine motor coordination and learned skilled motor acts.

### Qualitative

The psychologist identifies other motor disorders described in this chapter on the basis of qualitative data. These are obtained from an interview with the parent (or guardian), from school reports, and from clinical observation of the child.

**PARENT (GUARDIAN) INTERVIEW.** Information is obtained about a child's motor development and current motor skills. A distinction is made between a child's ability to perform a motor task spontaneously and his ability to perform the same task in response to a verbal command (see Appendix 2).

**SCHOOL REPORT.** The school report provides information about a child's motor performance (see Appendix 3).

**CLINICAL OBSERVATION.** Clinical observation provides information about the quality of a child's performance: (1) on standardized tests that require a motor act, (2) on age-appropriate motor tasks, and (3) in spontaneous behavior (see Appendix 4).

The diagnosis of motor disorders must include a referral to a neurologist for a neurological examination.

# REVIEW QUESTIONS

1. Fine motor coordination disturbances are typically associated with spinal cord dysfunction. True or False?
2. Name a feedback circuit that is critical to the modulation of motor activity.
3. Adequate coordination depends upon intact muscle tone and strength. True or False?
4. Where is the anterior horn located?
5. Tics, seen in children, are psychogenic in origin. True or False?
6. The peripheral nervous system is involved in control of human muscular activity. True or False?
7. Dyspraxia interferes with the learning of new motor skills. True or False?
8. What is the cortical dysfunction site associated with a perseveration disturbance?
9. Gille de la Tourette's syndrome is characterized by abnormal associated movements. True or False?
10. Define the two principal classes of motor function.
11. Fine motor and gross motor coordination disturbances usually coexist. True or False?
12. Overflow is a common phenomenon in children over ten years of age. True or False?
13. Name two motor systems.
14. The psychologist uses quantitative measurements to evaluate tone and strength. True or False?
15. Lower motor neurons originate in the cortex. True or False?

# 9

# READING DISORDERS

It has been estimated that some form of reading disorder affects as much as 20 percent of the school-aged population. It is not surprising, therefore, that difficulty in learning to read is frequently the presenting problem when a child is referred to a psychologist for an evaluation.

In order to diagnose a reading problem, one must evaluate the full range of factors that, singly and in concert, affect a child's ability to learn to read. In this chapter we summarize the historical background of the study of reading disorders; present the neuroanatomical basis of reading; define the clinical syndromes of reading disorders; outline the proposed subtypes of developmental reading disorders; and offer a guide to their diagnosis.

## HISTORICAL BACKGROUND

The earliest recorded description of an acquired reading disturbance dates back to 30 A.D., when a man was described who lost the ability to read following a blow to the head. He did not suffer any other cognitive disturbances. The next records of acquired isolated reading disturbances in adults date from the sixteenth century. Additional cases were recorded throughout the next three hundred years. During this time period, however, there was no attempt to correlate loss of reading with damage to a specific brain region.

In the late 1800's, associations between different types of reading problems and damage to focal brain areas were described. In one of the first of these reports, in 1877, it was proposed that the acquired reading disorder was a form of aphasia and was due to damage in the region of the angular gyrus, located at the temporal-parietal

FUNDAMENTALS OF CLINICAL CHILD NEUROPSYCHOLOGY


ISBN 0-8089-1910-5

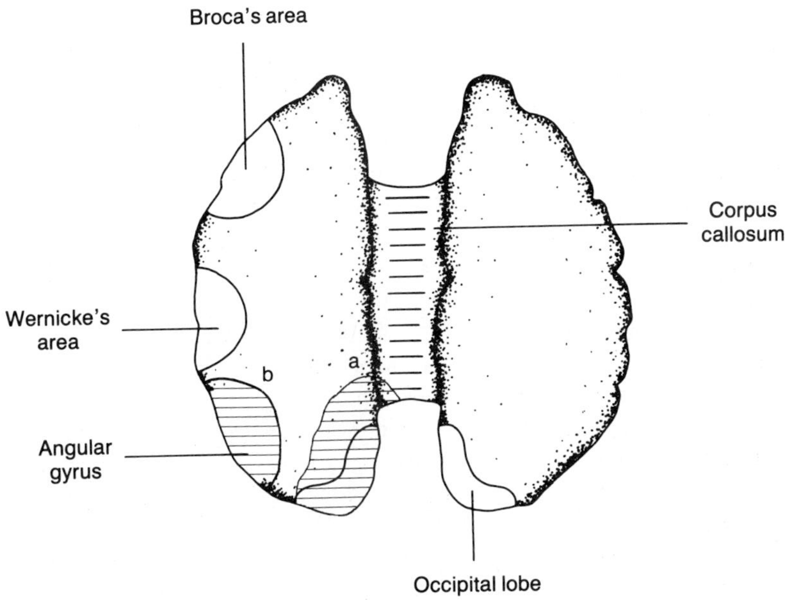


**Figure 9–1.** Schematic diagram of damaged areas of the brain associated with (a) alexia without agraphia and (b) alexia with agraphia. (Adopted with permission from Dyslexia: Neuropsychological theory, research, and clinical differentiation by G. Hynd and M. Cohen. Grune & Stratton, 1983.)

junction adjacent to the occipital lobe of the language-dominant hemisphere. This region was thereafter considered to be the memory center for words.

Major contributions to the theoretical conceptualization of reading disorders were made throughout the late nineteenth century. During this period, the two main subtypes of reading disorders were first recognized. Reading disorders were classified by: (1) the absence or (2) the presence of accompanying writing disorders. Reading disorders without accompanying writing disturbance were called *pure word blindness*. This type of disorder was considered to be the consequence of damage to the visual cortex (occipital lobe) in the language-dominant hemisphere in combination with a lesion in the posterior portion of the corpus callosum. It was thought that the lesion in the corpus callosum prevents the transfer of visual information from the intact, nondominant visual cortex to the dominant hemisphere, where it could be "read." In contrast, a reading disorder in which the ability to write was also lost (agraphia) was associated with a single lesion in the region of the angular gyrus of the dominant hemisphere. A schematic diagram of the damaged brain areas in (a) alexia without agraphia and (b) alexia with agraphia is presented in Figure 9-1.

Our understanding of reading disorders, associated cognitive deficits, and clinicoanatomical correlates has progressed rapidly in the period since World War II. Much of this knowledge has derived from significant advances in the neurosciences (e.g., development of the computerized transaxial tomography, or CT scan) and from new theoretical approaches to brain-behavior relationships. Most recently, there has been an increase in understanding of the reading process and reading failure as theoreticians and researchers have focused upon reading disturbances in children.

An early clinical description of a childhood reading disorder was published at the end of the nineteenth century. This report emphasized the similarities between the disturbances found in the child and those previously described in adults. It was not until the 1920's, however, that reading disorders in children were given a significant degree of attention. Research efforts at that time considered childhood reading problems to be a unitary disorder. Investigators sought a single etiology by comparing the reading skills of groups of disabled and normal readers.

Currently, it is proposed that reading disability in children does not represent a single homogeneous entity but that several syndromes exist. As a consequence, research in this area today focuses on the recognition and delineation of reading disorder subtypes. Such an approach is consistent with the fact that subtypes are well recognized among adults with acquired reading disorders. It is also consistent with current theories of brain-behavior relationships, which stress the complexity of cognitive and language functions.

## NEUROANATOMICAL BASIS OF READING

Reading, a higher mental process, may be conceptualized as depending upon a number of brain regions, each of which underlies a different aspect of the reading act. Some of the important brain regions vis à vis reading are as follows:

1. The occipital lobes of the right and left hemispheres process the visual input (words).
2. An association area within the language-dominant (usually the left) hemisphere translates the visual input into an auditory "message."
3. The receptive language region (Wernicke's area) of the dominant hemisphere "understands" the meaning of the message.
4. The motor region and expressive language (Broca's area) of the frontal lobe mediate scanning and verbalization of the message.

## CLINICAL READING DISORDER SYNDROMES

Reading disorders are divided into two major groups: (1) alexia, or acquired reading disorder, and (2) dyslexia, or developmental reading disorder. The term alexia refers to the loss of ability to read or the deterioration of reading competence. Alexia is the consequence of brain dysfunction suffered after reading skills have been learned. Dyslexia

**TABLE 9–1. SUMMARY OF SYNDROMES OF ALEXIA**

- I. Alexia without agraphia (pure alexia)
- II. Alexia with agraphia
  - A. Mild receptive language disturbance
  - B. Marked receptive language disturbance
  - C. Expressive language disturbance
  - D. Visual agnosia

refers to the failure to develop reading competence. Dyslexia is divided into three subgroups: (1) primary or specific, (2) symptomatic, and (3) secondary.

Primary dyslexia refers to a failure to develop reading competence (relative to level of intelligence) despite: (1) unimpaired vision and hearing, (2) motivation to learn, and (3) adequate educational experience. The disability is of constitutional origin and is due to subtle defects in higher cerebral functions. It is the most common form of dyslexia.

Symptomatic dyslexia refers to reading disability resulting from cerebral dysfunction that is the consequence of very early insult to the brain, for example, perinatal brain damage.

Secondary dyslexia is a rare result of extremely adverse environmental, emotional, and/or general health factors.

## ALEXIA

As described earlier, initial understanding of reading disability was based on the case histories of acquired reading difficulty in brain damaged adults. As noted, alexia was divided into two classes, defined by (1) the absence or (2) the presence of a concurrent writing disorder (agraphia). Table 9–1 summarizes the alexia subtypes, which are discussed below.

### *Alexia without Agraphia*

Alexia without agraphia, or pure alexia, is relatively rare. It is characterized by impairment in the comprehension of written language, both single words and text. Copying ability is impaired but writing and spelling are not. Oral language is normal, although mild word finding difficulty (anomia) affecting objects and colors may exist. Arithmetic calculation may be impaired.

Alexia without agraphia is a disconnection syndrome. A disconnection syndrome is a disorder that is the result of damage to either: (1) cortical association fibers, which connect cortical regions within a hemisphere, or (2) commissural fibers, which connect regions in the two cortical hemispheres. Alexia without agraphia is classified as a disconnection syndrome, since it is due to a lesion in the dominant occipital lobe in conjunction with a lesion in the posterior portion of the corpus callosum.

### *Alexia with Agraphia*

Alexia with agraphia is the most frequently encountered form of acquired reading disorder. It has been associated with four types of disturbance: (1) mild receptive language disturbance, (2) marked receptive language disturbance, (3) expressive language disturbance, and (4) visual agnosia.

**MILD RECEPTIVE LANGUAGE DISTURBANCE.** Alexia with agraphia in which receptive language disturbance is mild and oral language is spared is characterized by impairment in reading and in the full range of writing skills. Naming and calculation are mildly impaired.

This disorder is usually associated with dysfunction of the dominant angular gyrus.

**MARKED RECEPTIVE LANGUAGE DISTURBANCE.** Alexia with agraphia associated with severe receptive aphasia is characterized by severe impairment in the reading of letters, words, or both. Writing is always diffusely impaired, and an arithmetic disorder (acalculia) is commonly present.

Dysfunction in the dominant posterior temporal lobe is usually associated with this disorder.

**EXPRESSIVE LANGUAGE DISTURBANCE.** When alexia with agraphia is a component of expressive aphasia, the recognition and production of written language are impaired. Reading is especially impaired for relational words (e.g., *before, under*) and for words that serve as grammatical markers (e.g., *but, and*). Words that have high semantic value (e.g., *table, car*) are read with less difficulty. Eye movements are also impaired.

This disorder is typically related to dysfunction in the frontal lobe of the dominant hemisphere.

**VISUAL AGNOSIA.** This reading-writing disorder is conceptualized as a feature of visual agnosia (see Chapter 7). Visual recognition and the ability to reproduce complex forms are impaired.

Right parietal lobe dysfunction is usually implicated in this disorder.

## Dyslexia

Dyslexia is now recognized as a heterogeneous disorder, and attempts have been made to identify dyslexia subtypes on the basis of neuropsychological and neurolinguistic models.

Proponents of the neuropsychological model described such groups as the auditory-linguistic, the visual-spatial perceptual, and the motor discoordination.

The neurolinguistic school has described phonological, deep, and surface dyslexia subgroups.

Representative dyslexia subtypes are summarized in Table 9–2 and discussed below.

### *Neuropsychological Subtypes*

**AUDITORY-LINGUISTIC** Auditory-linguistic dyslexia is characterized by

**TABLE 9–2. REPRESENTATIVE SUBTYPES OF DYSLEXIA**

I. Neuropsychological
  A. Auditory-linguistic
  B. Visual-spatial perceptual
  C. Motor discoordination
II. Psycholinguistic
  A. Phonological
  B. Deep
  C. Surface

generally compromised development of language functions. For example, a child with this syndrome may have difficulty retrieving verbal labels or may show poor discrimination of speech sounds. Learning letter-sound associations and blending phonemes into words are difficult. Reading and spelling performance are seriously deficient. The child's functioning in arithmetic may also be poor. Other deficits associated with this syndrome include poor motor coordination and difficulty in speech articulation. This is the most common deficit pattern, and it occurs most frequently in boys.

**VISUAL-SPATIAL PERCEPTUAL.** A child with this type of reading disturbance has no language deficits but has impaired visual-spatial memory and impaired visual perception. Letters and words that are physically similar (e.g., *m–w, them–then*) are often confused. This deficit appears with equal frequency in boys and girls.

**MOTOR DISCOORDINATION.** This dyslexia is characterized by oromotor apraxia and difficulty with sound blending. Reading tends to be limited to a sight vocabulary. There is often difficulty in writing, due to poor fine motor skills.

### *Neurolinguistic Subtypes*

**PHONOLOGICAL.** This dyslexia is characterized by difficulty forming letter-sound associations. Familiar words can be read, but there is difficulty reading function words (e.g., *and, but*) and nonsense words (e.g., *tev*). The meaning of words is understood.

**DEEP.** This is described as a rare form of phonological dyslexia in which the misread word has a relationship to the target word. For example, "red" may be read for the target word "blue." Familiar words are read well. Concrete and frequently appearing words are read more accurately than abstract words. Comprehension is not affected.

**SURFACE.** In this subtype, words that do not follow phonological rules are troublesome. Long words are read less easily than short words. The individual is able to apply phonological rules well. He is able to decode nonsense words well. Overall comprehension is poor.

## DIAGNOSIS OF READING DISORDERS

The current diagnostic and statistical manual and the current research literature provide guidelines for the diagnosis of reading disorders.

Our approach to the diagnosis of reading disorders relies on the integration of quantitative and qualitative information. The first step in the diagnostic task is delineation of the reading process. The diagnostic procedure requires assessment of a child's strengths and deficits in the various subskills required for reading competence.

### Delineation of the Reading Act

It is common to conceptualize reading competence as depending upon the ability to perform two tasks. The first task is that of decoding, or conversion of the written word into oral language. The second task is that of comprehension, or understanding the meaning of the written message. Typically, a diagnostic evaluation is limited to measures of performance on decoding and comprehension tasks. In our view, diagnosis of a reading disorder depends upon a more extensive delineation and assessment of these two aspects of the reading act.

#### *DECODING*

The reading act depends upon two strategies: the phonetic and the sight. The phonetic strategy consists of: (1) recall of letter-sound (grapheme-phoneme) associations and (2) blending of individual sounds to create short words or syllables and blending of syllables to create longer words. The sight approach is based upon recognition of visual word patterns.

The steps underlying the act of decoding include a number of subskills:

1. First, a child's senses must be intact. He must possess a sufficient level of auditory, visual, and somatosensory acuity to allow adequate reception of oral and visual information.
2. Beyond acuity, adequate perceptual discrimination of the stimuli is required. A child must be able to make gross and fine discriminations in the visual, auditory, and somatosensory modalities.
3. For letter-sound and word-label associations that are taught directly, a child must be able to make the necessary visual-auditory associations.
4. When letter-sound associations are not taught directly, a child must be able to segment the individual sounds within an orally presented word and to associate each one with a letter.
5. A child must also be capable of conditional learning. Letter-sound associations often depend upon surrounding letters (e.g., *c* in *cat* compared to *c* in *fancy*). He must be able to produce the sound appropriate to the context.
6. A child must also be able to shift between modalities. The process of decoding requires a repeated shift of attention between visual and auditory (letter and sound, or word and label) stimuli.

7. After recalling the letter-sound associations, but before they are blended, auditory sequential memory functions come into play. A child must be able to remember the correct sequence of sounds to be blended. If syllabication is required, he must be able to remember the string of syllables to be combined, in their correct order.
8. A child must be able to blend sounds.
9. A consistent and smooth left-to-right scanning and work pattern must be maintained.
10. A child's sight reading depends upon visual sequential or visual-spatial memory functions. He must be able to remember the visual array of the target word. He must also be able to form the visual-auditory association between target word and label.
11. A child must be able to shift between phonetic and sight strategies as needed.
12. In oral reading, expressive language and speech functions must be intact.

#### *COMPREHENSION*

In our framework, underlying the task of understanding the meaning of the written message, the following subskills are noteworthy:

1. A child must be able to decode the written word accurately. All the subskills that are required for the decoding process must be functioning adequately.
2. In reading sentences and paragraphs, a child's auditory memory system must be capable of performing multiple memory tasks in parallel and sequentially. A child must be able to use the auditory sequential memory system at the phoneme level to decode individual words and also at the linguistic level to remember the content of the message as the words are decoded.
3. Language skills must be such that a child is able to grasp the meaning of individual words and to combine the individual words so as to grasp the whole message.
4. Visual markings of written language (e.g., quotation marks) must be understood.
5. A child must be able to maintain his place on a line and on a page.

## ASSESSMENT OF READING COMPETENCE AND READING SUBSKILLS

The diagnosis of reading disorders requires the integration of quantitative and qualitative information. Quantitative assessment is based on a child's performance on standardized tests of reading competence and reading subskills. Qualitative information is obtained from a variety of sources (e.g., reports from parents or guardians and school, special clinical procedures). Representative quantitative and qualitative measures of reading competence and reading subskills are presented in Appendices 11 and 12.

### *Quantitative Assessment*

#### READING COMPETENCE

***Decoding.*** A number of standardized tests of decoding are available. These tests assess a child's ability to decode words singly and within the context of sentences and paragraphs.

***Comprehension.*** There are standardized tests of reading comprehension that involve oral and silent reading of paragraphs and others that involve oral and silent reading of single words. Both assess a child's ability to understand the meaning of a written message through his answers to questions about the reading material.

**READING SUBSKILLS.** Standardized tests are available for such reading subskills as perceptual discrimination, letter-sound associations, sound blending, and memory functions, as well as for the global abilities of language and general intelligence that impact on reading performance.

### *Qualitative Assessment*

The qualitative information used to obtain a diagnosis of a child's reading disorder includes data gathered from the following:

**PARENT (GUARDIAN) INTERVIEW.** Information about the child's school history is obtained. Special note is made of reading and of spelling performance.

Developmental and medical histories of the child are obtained. Familial patterns of developmental disorders are noted (see Appendix 2).

**SCHOOL REPORT.** The school report supplies information on a child's academic achievement as well as on behavioral and motivational factors that might be affecting the learning process (see Appendix 3).

**CLINICAL OBSERVATION.** Information about a child's reading competence and reading subskills are obtained by observing the quality of his: (1) performance on standardized tests, (2) performance on age-appropriate informal tests, and (3) spontaneous verbalizations and behavior. The psychologist must note not only right and wrong answers but the nature of the errors. He should also note whether decoding is done smoothly or with many false starts and whether or not decoding is accurate. Because poor performance on a comprehension test may reflect a child's preoccupation with inner thoughts rather than failure to understand a written message, motivation to do well and attention to the reading task are noted. A true comprehension disorder ( in which ability to decode is intact but ability to understand meaning is impaired), is very rare (see Appendix 4).

## REVIEW QUESTIONS

1. Alexia refers to a loss of ability to read by previously competent readers. True or False?
2. Reading disorders in children are rare. True or False?
3. A child's inability to learn to read is always the result of emotional or environmental factors. True or False?
4. Researchers have always been interested in developmental reading disorders. True or False?

5. What is the difference between alexia and dyslexia?
6. Alexia is divided into two major subtypes. What are they?
7. Alexia never occurs in conjunction with aphasia. True or False?
8. Alexia with agraphia is a disconnection syndrome. True or False?
9. The majority of acquired reading disorders are associated with damage to the right hemisphere. True or False?
10. Define *pure word blindness*.
11. The corpus callosum plays an important role in reading. True or False?
12. Describe the two strategies used in the act of reading.
13. Name three decoding subskills.
14. Dyslexia is divided into two major subtypes. True or False?
15. Performance on a standardized test of decoding is a sufficient measure of reading competence. True or False?

# 10

# WRITING DISORDERS

A large proportion of the children who are referred to a psychologist have writing and/or spelling problems. Unlike reading problems, which may be rather elusive, writing and spelling problems are intrinsically difficult to conceal and therefore relatively easy to recognize. Determining the nature of the problem, however, usually requires careful probing, because a large number of neuropsychological factors affect a child's ability to learn to produce written language.

In this chapter, we present an overview of writing disorders. We give the historical background of the study of writing problems; discuss the neuroanatomical basis of writing; define and discuss the clinical writing disorder syndromes, describe the errors associated with developmental writing problems; and delineate the tasks involved in the diagnosis of writing disorders.

## HISTORICAL BACKGROUND

Even a cursory review of the brain-behavior literature reveals that writing disturbances have been of interest to many investigators for over a century. First described in the 1850's, writing disturbances were initially envisioned (in the absence of any brain-behavior data or any inferences regarding brain-behavior correlates) in terms of two basic groups.

The first group involved motor disorders. In this category were patients who had difficulty in the very act of producing written language. This was considered to reflect a breakdown in the association between the sound image of a word and the neural impulses that activate the preferred hand to produce the word's graphic representation.

The second group involved language disorders. In this group were individuals who

FUNDAMENTALS OF CLINICAL CHILD NEUROPSYCHOLOGY

ISBN 0-8089-1910-5

were able to produce single written letters but had difficulty in producing a correctly spelled word. This problem was considered to reflect either of two possible disturbances: (1) deficient ability to form or recall verbal images or (2) deficient ability to associate those verbal images with visual images (their graphic representations).

In the 1870's, there was a shift in thinking about writing disturbances. During this period, it became generally accepted that they always reflected a language problem. Researchers began to hypothesize that writing disorders were associated with a defect in the left temporal area of the brain, which underlies language functions. Moreover, it was suggested that any brain defect that spares language function also spares writing functions.

Beginning in the 1880's, papers began to appear that described acquired writing disorders in adults who had no language problems. It was hypothesized that the loss of writing skills in such individuals was due to a brain deficit that affected either motor output alone or visual-spatial perception alone. In the former instance, the writing problem would be the result of inability to produce the movements necessary for writing. In the latter, writing problems would be the result of inability to perceive or remember the spatial aspects of visual graphic images. In either case, the notion of the subordination of writing to auditory language functions was challenged.

Today, writing is understood to depend upon underlying language functions, visual-spatial functions, and their integration with graphomotor functions. The present understanding of writing disturbances takes into account adult clinical data, an appreciation of the subskills involved in writing, the brain regions that underlie these skills, and the differing requirements of specific writing tasks. This understanding, parenthetically, has contributed to the current view of writing as a particularly complex and vulnerable function, one that is especially sensitive to subtle alteration in brain processes.

## NEUROANATOMICAL BASIS OF WRITING

Writing skills depend upon a number of brain regions, each of which underlies a different component of writing competence. Some of the most important functions of the brain regions vis à vis writing can be summarized as follows:

1. The dominant (usually left) temporal region mediates speech reception and discrimination.
2. The dominant temporal lobe governs maintenance of the speech sound sequence for the analysis and production of written material.
3. Association areas of the dominant hemisphere are responsible for sound-letter and whole word-visual image conversion.
4. The dominant parietal lobe stores information about the visual-kinesthetic features of letters.
5. The frontal area controls motor programming and production of verbal output (oral spelling) and graphic output (written spelling).
6. The posterior right hemisphere mediates spatial orientation on the page, spacing within and between words, and letter form.

**TABLE 10-1. SYNDROMES OF AGRAPHIA**

I. Pure agraphia
II. Agraphia associated with aphasia
  A. Receptive aphasia
  B. Expressive aphasia
  C. Conduction aphasia
III. Spatial agraphia
IV. Apraxic agraphia

7. The prefrontal area controls the switching between auditory and visual representations of linguistic materials that occurs during writing, and also sustains attention to the writing task.

## CLINICAL WRITING DISORDER SYNDROMES

Writing disorders are divided into two major categories: (1) agraphia, or acquired writing disorder, which is the consequence of brain dysfunction that occurs after writing skills have been learned; and (2) dysgraphia, or developmental writing disorder, which refers to the failure to develop writing competence. *Dysgraphia* should not be confused with *dysorthographia*, a term that may be generically applied to all cases of written spelling disorder. Dysorthographia may be seen in many of the writing disorders described in this chapter.

### Agraphia

Agraphia is usually divided into four categories: (1) pure agraphia, (2) agraphia associated with aphasia, (3) spatial agraphia, and (4) apraxic agraphia. Table 10-1 summarizes the classes of agraphia, discussed below.

#### *Pure Agraphia*

Pure agraphia is quite rare. It is characterized by poor written spelling ability in the presence of intact reading and writing skills plus intact oral spelling ability. An individual with this disorder may or may not retain the ability to spell with letter blocks.

The underlying defect in pure agraphia remains a topic of considerable debate. It has been associated with dysfunction in the dominant frontal region, the dominant parietal region, and the connections between these two areas.

#### *Agraphia Associated with Aphasia*

Agraphia associated with aphasia (language dysfunction) is the most common type of agraphia. Three different writing-language problems have been described: (1) agraphia associated with receptive language disturbance, (2) agraphia associated with expressive language disturbance, and (3) agraphia associated with conduction aphasia (see Chapter 4, Table 4–1).

**AGRAPHIA ASSOCIATED WITH RECEPTIVE APHASIA.** In agraphia with receptive language disturbance, spelling in spontaneous writing and to dictation is seriously compromised. However, ability to copy written language is relatively intact. Two subtypes of agraphia with receptive aphasia exist, in which either (1) speech discrimination or (2) language comprehension is impaired.

When discrimination of speech sounds is impaired, as in *pure word deafness* (in adults) and verbal auditory agnosia (in children), spelling is less disturbed in spontaneous writing than in writing to dictation. When impaired comprehension is the primary receptive language deficit, the effects on writing are different. Spelling in spontaneous writing is seriously disturbed, while spelling to dictation is relatively spared. In writing to dictation, real words are produced with many fewer errors than nonsense words (e.g., *ton* vs. *tob*).

The location of the brain defect in these two subtypes is usually the same as that implicated in the associated receptive language disorder, namely, the dominant temporal area.

**AGRAPHIA ASSOCIATED WITH EXPRESSIVE APHASIA.** When agraphia occurs with an expressive language disturbance, an individual's copying remains intact, but spontaneous writing and writing to dictation are impaired. In writing to dictation, production of real words is better than production of nonsense syllables. Though individual letters can be well produced, the quality of graphomotor productions deteriorates at the word level. An individual with this disorder always has seriously impaired spelling. When expressive language disturbance is characterized by agrammatical speech, agraphia is generally characterized by telegraphic writing.

This writing disorder is usually associated with a defect in the dominant frontal region that underlies expressive language.

**AGRAPHIA ASSOCIATED WITH CONDUCTION APHASIA.** The third class of aphasia-related writing disorders is associated with a disturbance in verbal repetition (called conduction aphasia in adults). In this disorder, spontaneous writing and writing to dictation are impaired, while copying is intact. Individual letters are well formed, but written productions deteriorate at the word level. Overwriting is common. An individual with this disorder can write real words to dictation better than nonsense syllables. Written and oral spelling are impaired. In writing, there are omissions and substitutions of letters. Paraphasias (word substitutions) are common. Words that are phonetically similar are confused and substituted for one another. Well-practiced and overlearned words (e.g., name, address) are produced accurately, however.

The underlying dysfunction in this syndrome is usually the same as that associated with conduction aphasia.

### *Spatial Agraphia*

Spatial agraphia is characterized by defects in the spatial features of written graphic productions. The writing of an individual with this disorder is characterized by

**TABLE 10-2. ERRORS MADE BY CHILDREN WITH A WRITING DISORDER**

1. Linguistic errors
2. Dysphonetic spelling
3. Dyseidetic spelling
4. Letter rotation, inversion, or both
5. Reversed letter sequence, syllable inversion, or both
6. Mirror writing
7. Spatial disorganization
8. Poor handwriting
9. Defective written spelling
10. Perseveration, substitution, and/or omission of letters, syllables, and/or words

irregular spacing between letters, syllables, and words, and it typically slants toward the bottom or top of the page. There is a perseverative quality to the written letters. For example, many letters have noticeable extra strokes. In addition, such an individual's writing may occupy only one half of a page—most often, the right half.

In most cases, spatial agraphia is attributed to posterior right hemisphere dysfunction.

### *Apraxic Agraphia*

Apraxic agraphia is characterized by poor writing and poor spelling. An individual with this disorder performs poorly when copying, when writing spontaneously, and when writing to dictation, although the syntax of written language remains unimpaired. Even spelling with letter blocks is never entirely spared, though it often remains stronger than written spelling. Apraxic agraphia is often associated with disturbances of oral language.

This disorder is commonly associated with dysfunction of the parietal region opposite the dominant hand.

## Dysgraphia

To date, few significant efforts have been made to isolate and delineate developmental writing disorders. However, it has been shown clearly that these disorders are characterized by several different kinds of errors. Disturbances in writing ability can involve: (1) a breakdown of the linguistic features of language that is not apparent in oral communication, (2) inaccuracies in the spatial features of graphic letter or word productions, and (3) poor execution of the graphomotor act. The types of errors commonly made by children with writing problems are summarized in Table 10-2 and described below.

1. Linguistic errors. These are errors in the syntax and semantics of written language that are not apparent in spoken language. Punctuation rules are not applied.
2. Dysphonetic spelling. Written words are not recognizable because of lack of

phonetic correspondence to the target word. There is difficulty writing from dictation and spontaneously. Copying ability is unimpaired. Well-practiced words are written correctly.

3. Dyseidetic spelling. Misspelled words are recognizable because the spelling is phonetically correct (e.g., nature-nacher). Spelling of phonetically irregular words (e.g., give) is especially poor.

4. Letter rotation, inversion, or both. Although young children often reverse asymmetrical letters such as *b* and *d*, when this pattern persists beyond the age of seven years, it is cause for concern.

5. Reversed letter sequence, syllable inversion, or both. This error pattern involves incorrect letter sequences (e.g., once-ocne). Both oral and written spelling are impaired.

6. Mirror writing. In mirror writing, words are correctly spelled and letters are correctly formed but written backward (e.g., in-ni).

7. Spatial disorganization. These errors resemble those seen in spatial agraphia (see above): (a) neglect of the left side of a word or the left side of the paper that is being written upon, (b) lines of writing that slope toward the top or bottom of the page, (c) difficulty going from the right end of a line to the left (or beginning) end of the next line, and (d) poor spacing of letters, syllables, and words.

8. Poor handwriting. Writing is illegible. Oral spelling is intact. Copying is less impaired than spontaneous writing or writing to dictation.

9. Defective written spelling. Oral spelling is intact, but there is an inability to correctly write the same words that are spelled orally. Writing to dictation and spontaneously are impaired but copying written words is not affected. Handwriting is unimpaired. This error pattern is extremely rare.

10. Perseveration, substitution, and/or omission of letters, syllables, and/or words. This type of writing pattern involves intact spelling subskills that are not used consistently. As a consequence, repetitions, substitutions, and omissions of letters, syllables, and words occur sporadically throughout a piece of writing. This type of error pattern is rare.

## DIAGNOSIS OF WRITING DISORDERS

The current diagnostic and statistical manual and the current research literature provide guidelines for the diagnosis of writing disorders.

Our approach to the diagnosis of a writing disorder is based upon the integration of quantitative and qualitative information. The first and crucial step in this process is a delineation of the writing act.

### Delineation of the Writing Act

In our view, writing competence depends upon an individual's ability to perform a number of discrete tasks, notably: (1) conversion, in which the orally presented word is analyzed and converted into a mental visual image; (2) translation, in which the visual image is translated into a graphic or oral production; and (3) integration, in which an internal message is generated spontaneously and encoded into a written one, a process requiring fully integrated language subskills.

**CONVERSION.** Conversion of an oral word stimulus into a visual mental image is accomplished by two strategies: the phonetic and the sight. The phonetic strategy consists of: (a) segmenting of orally presented words into individual speech sounds and (b) recall of sound-letter (phoneme-grapheme) associations. The sight approach is based on recall of visual word patterns. These strategies rely upon many subskills such as:

1. A child must have adequate auditory, visual, and somatosensory acuity.
2. He must have adequate auditory, visual and somatosensory discrimination ability.
3. He must be able to segment a word into individual speech sounds (phonemes) and to form sound-letter associations.
4. He must be able to recall the sound-letter associations for each individual speech sound within the word.
5. For words that cannot be spelled phonetically, a child must be able to recall the appropriate visual word image.
6. He must be able to recall special spelling rules.
7. He must be able to shift back and forth between the auditory and visual modalities.
8. He must be able to sustain a consistent work pattern (left-to-right).
9. Fluent writing depends upon continuous addition of phonetically analyzed words into the word image memory store.
10. A child must be able to shift between phonetic and sight strategies as needed.

**TRANSLATION.** Translation of a visual image into a graphic or oral production depends notably upon:

1. Activation of a kinesthetic schema by the visual image.
2. Development of motor programs based on kinesthetic information.
3. Activation of the appropriate complex motor programs for written or oral spelling.
4. Initiation of motor commands.
5. Production of a written or oral spelling.

**INTEGRATION.** Spontaneous production of chains of written words that adhere to the basic rules of semantics (word meaning) and syntax (grammar) involves intact oral language skills and their utilization during the act of writing.

## Assessment of Writing Competence and Writing Subskills

Various types of writing tasks depend to different degrees upon language, visual-spatial, and motor skills. For example, copying written words depends most heavily upon visual-spatial skills and least upon language skills.

The diagnosis of writing disorders entails the combined use of quantitative and qualitative data obtained in different types of writing tasks. Both writing competence and writing subskills are assessed. Quantitative measures are derived from a child's performance on standardized tests of writing competence and writing subskills. Qualitative information is obtained from many different sources (e.g., reports from parents and schools, special clinical procedures). A summary of commonly used quantitative and qualitative measures of writing competence and writing subskills is presented in Appendices 13 and 14.

### *Quantitative*

**WRITING COMPETENCE.** There are standardized measures of writing competence that examine written spelling, punctuation and capitalization, spontaneous writing (word usage and theme), and handwriting.

**WRITING SUBSKILLS.** There are standardized tests of such subskills as: visual, auditory, and somatosensory discrimination and both auditory and visual short-term memory. Fine motor coordination and graphomotor functions are assessed quantitatively, as are language functions and verbal intelligence.

### *Qualitative*

The qualitative assessment of a child's writing competence and writing subskills utilizes data obtained from an interview with the parent (guardian), from school report, and from clinical observation of the child.

**PARENT (GUARDIAN) INTERVIEW.** Information is obtained about a child's writing skills. The distinction between handwriting per se and written and oral spelling is stressed. In addition to developmental history, the psychologist obtains medical and family histories. Familial patterns of writing disorders are noted (see Appendix 2).

**SCHOOL REPORT.** The school report gives information about a child's writing competence and subskills and written spelling (see Appendix 3).

**CLINICAL OBSERVATION.** Clinical observation provides information about the quality of a child's performance (1) on standardized tests of writing, (2) on age-appropriate writing tasks, and (3) in spontaneous writing. This information is vital to an assessment of his writing competence (see Appendix 4).

In evaluating a child's writing, special care must be given to the examination of qualitative differences between:

1. Practiced and unpracticed written words.
2. Writing samples obtained in different writing tasks such as: copying, writing to dictation, and spontaneous writing (copying involves writing with a model present; dictation involves writing specific letters or words that are presented orally; spontaneous writing involves writing whatever you want to write).

A child's written productions must always be evaluated in light of his oral productions, both those made in response to direct questions or on command, and those offered spontaneously.

Whenever a child presents with poor writing, special attention must be given to his fine motor skills. Fine motor skills must be intact in order to make a diagnosis of dysgraphia.

## REVIEW QUESTIONS

1. Describe characteristic features of pure agraphia.
2. Describe typical errors in dysphonetic spelling.
3. Before the diagnosis of dysgraphia can be made, what is the most important disturbance that must be ruled out?
4. Writing disorders are always subordinate to auditory language problems. True or False?
5. Describe mirror writing.
6. What are the features of agraphia with expressive aphasia?
7. What brain area is implicated when writing is poorly organized on the page?
8. Beyond what age are letter reversals a cause for concern?
9. Writing competence depends upon the complex interaction of what three functions?
10. Dysphonetic spellers do not have a problem in copying written words. True or False?
11. Spelling errors that yield recognizable words point to the use of which spelling strategy?
12. Name the brain area that is disturbed when written letters are poorly spaced.
13. All dysgraphics have fine motor disturbances. True or False?
14. Children with language disorders always have writing problems. True or False?
15. Children with fine motor disorders always have writing problems. True or False?

# 11

# ARITHMETIC DISORDERS

Teachers and parents often seek the help of a psychologist in obtaining a better understanding of a child's difficulties in mastering arithmetic skills. It must be recognized at the outset that problems in arithmetic competence may reflect a range of disturbances such as: a global defect (e.g., poor intelligence), a specific defect (e.g., visual-spatial disturbance), or a true arithmetic disorder.

In this chapter, we summarize the background literature on arithmetic disorders; present the neuroanatomical basis of arithmetic performance; overview the clinical arithmetic disorder syndromes, including arithmetic disorders in children; and present a guide to the diagnosis of developmental arithmetic disorders.

## HISTORICAL BACKGROUND

The earliest reports of arithmetic disorders date back to the late 1800's. These reports involved adult patients who had suffered brain injuries that primarily affected language functions but also involved serious loss or deterioration of the ability to calculate. The early reports encouraged investigators at the time to conclude that calculation problems were always associated with, if not caused by, language problems.

In the early 1900's, it was recognized that some forms of arithmetic disability exist in the absence of an explicit language disturbance. As a result, acquired arithmetic disorders were divided into two groups: primary and secondary. Primary arithmetic problems are those that are not attributable to any broader underlying disturbance in mental function, such as language disability, poor memory, or inadequate intelligence. Secondary arithmetic disorders are those that exist within the context of such an underlying disturbance. Over the last thirty years, a number of different classification systems have been proposed. To date, no one system has been widely accepted.

FUNDAMENTALS OF CLINICAL CHILD NEUROPSYCHOLOGY

ISBN 0-8089-1910-5

**TABLE 11-1. SYNDROMES OF ACALCULIA**

| | |
|---|---|
| I. | Primary acalculia |
| II. | Acalculia associated with alexia and/or agraphia for numbers |
| III. | Acalculia secondary to visual-spatial disturbance |

Childhood arithmetic disorders have not received much investigative attention. An early clinical description of a childhood arithmetic disturbance was published in the 1930's. Since that time, case studies and retrospective studies have dominated the sparse literature in this area.

## NEUROANATOMICAL BASIS OF ARITHMETIC

Arithmetic competence is based on a functional system formed by the interaction of a number of cortical regions, including:

1. The right hemisphere mediates visual-spatial organization.
2. The occipital lobes mediate discrimination of written numbers and operation signs.
3. The left parietal lobe mediates sequencing abilities.
4. The dominant temporal lobe mediates memory of number series, number facts (e.g., 4 + 1 = 5), and subvocal functions involved in word problem solving.
5. Higher association areas of the dominant hemisphere mediate the comprehension of numerical concepts and operations and the decoding and comprehension of word problems.
6. The frontal area mediates problem-solving skills and is crucial to production of written and oral arithmetic performance.

## CLINICAL ARITHMETIC DISORDER SYNDROMES

Disturbances in the ability to perform numerical tasks are divided into two major classes: (1) acalculia, or acquired arithmetic disorder, the result of brain injury suffered after arithmetic skills have been mastered; and (2) dyscalculia, or developmental arithmetic disorder, which refers to the failure to develop arithmetic competence.

### Acalculia

Acquired arithmetic disorders are commonly divided into three categories: (1) primary acalculia, (2) acalculia associated with alexia and/or agraphia for numbers, and (3) acalculia secondary to visual-spatial disturbance (see Table 11–1).

### *Primary Acalculia*

In a primary arithmetic disorder, difficulty in performing numerical calculations is not associated with a language or visual-spatial disturbance. The arithmetic problem is a loss of understanding of the meaning or concept of numbers. In addition to not being able to perform arithmetic computations, an individual with this disorder has a hard time with mathematical estimations (e.g., how long is your arm?). Calculation difficulties are equally severe whether numbers are presented visually or orally. Word problems pose as many difficulties as calculation problems, and difficulties are equally severe whether the presentation is visual or oral.

Primary acalculia is usually associated with left hemisphere dysfunction. In rare cases, it has also been reported in adult patients with right hemisphere dysfunction.

### *Acalculia with Alexia and/or Agraphia for Numbers*

This disorder is often referred to as aphasic acalculia. An individual with such a disorder tends to misname written numbers and to have difficulty coming up with the names of numbers when speaking. Reading and writing of numbers are also impaired. Substitutions involving numbers that sound alike or look alike are common. He may have difficulty with the names of the calculation operations (e.g., addition) that are associated with the graphic symbols (e.g., +). Arithmetic word problems pose even greater difficulties. These difficulties are equally severe whether the problems are presented in writing or orally. The ability to calculate is preserved.

Most often, the underlying dysfunction in this type of acalculia is localized to either left or bilateral brain regions.

### *Acalculia Secondary to Visual-Spatial Disturbance*

An individual with acalculia secondary to visual-spatial disturbance often makes errors stemming from neglect of the left side of the visual field when reading and/or writing numbers. There is also evidence of visual drift in writing numbers. Errors involving the reading and writing of multidigit numbers, the alignment of number columns, and the place-holding value of numbers are common. Such individuals typically lack awareness of calculation errors and as a result have poor ability to recognize and correct them. However, an individual with this type of acalculia has no special difficulty with dictated calculation or word problems which can be solved by means of mental calculation.

Brain dysfunction in this disorder is usually confined to the right parietal region. In some cases of spatial acalculia, bilateral dysfunction has been reported.

## Dyscalculia

The arithmetic errors described in each of the three acalculia categories have all

**TABLE 11-2. ERRORS MADE BY CHILDREN WITH AN ARITHMETIC DISORDER**

1. Number sequence errors
2. Basic concept errors
3. Number comprehension errors
4. Finger counting errors
5. Written number inversions, rotations, or both
6. Misalignment of numbers
7. Spatial disorganization
8. Inappropriate work pattern
9. Linguistic errors
10. Perseveration errors

been described in children. In children, these errors may be seen in the same clusters as in adults, but they may also be seen singly and in a variety of different combinations, cutting across all of the acalculia subtypes. The error types may reflect disturbances in the three main features of arithmetic competence: (1) number comprehension and counting, (2) ability to calculate, and (3) ability to solve numerical word problems. Some common types of errors made by children with an arithmetic disorder are summarized in Table 11–2 and discussed below.

1. Number sequence errors. These errors are apparent in written and/or oral performance.

2. Basic concept errors. These errors involve basic concepts of position and order (e.g., *before, after, in front, behind)* or size and quantity (e.g., *smaller, larger*; *fewer, more).*

3. Number comprehension errors. These are errors in the "practical" skills that rely upon an understanding of number concepts (e.g., tell time, make change) and numerical estimations. Place value confusions are common.

4. Finger counting errors. These are errors in counting fingers to obtain answers to basic calculation problems (e.g., 2 + 3, 4 - 1).

5. Written number inversions, rotations, or both. Calculation errors are commonly associated with the inaccurately written numbers which characterize this error pattern.

6. Misalignment of numbers. This error pattern involves difficulty organizing numbers in written calculation. Misalignment of numbers in columns, errors in addition with carrying, in subtraction with borrowing, and in multiplication and division are common.

7. Spatial disorganization. In this type of problem, a child misplaces decimal points and thus has difficulty calculating percentages as well as converting decimals into percentages and vice versa. He also has difficulty with fractions. One half of the visual field is usually distorted or neglected. Reading and writing of numbers may be affected. Such reading and writing errors are confined to the affected visual field. Writing is characterized by spatial drift (i.e., writing slopes toward the top or bottom of the page). Word problems that can be solved mentally pose no special difficulty.

8. Inappropriate work pattern. These errors are characterized by use of an inappropriate work pattern in numerical calculations (e.g.,left to right for multidigit addi-

tion, subtraction, and multiplication). Word problems that can be solved mentally pose no difficulty.

9. Linguistic errors. This type of error pattern involves misnaming of written numbers and number labels when speaking. Difficulty learning the names of the calculation operations and the association between the graphic signs and the operation names (once the latter are learned) is common. Arithmetic word problems that require both understanding of the linguistic content and selection of an appropriate numerical operation pose the greatest difficulty.

10. Perseveration errors. This error pattern involves failure to shift from one operation to another (e.g., addition to subtraction) or responding to a word problem with the number last heard or used.

## DIAGNOSIS OF ARITHMETIC DISORDERS

The current diagnostic and statistical manual and the current literature provide guidelines for the diagnosis of arithmetic disorders.

Our approach to the diagnosis of a developmental arithmetic disorder requires the integration of a range of quantitative and qualitative information. The initial step in defining the information that is needed depends upon a careful delineation of arithmetic subskills.

### Delination of Arithmetic Subskills

We conceptualize arithmetic competence as depending upon the ability to perform a number of tasks. These can be divided into three broad categories: (1) number comprehension and counting, (2) calculation, and (3) numerical word problem solving.

**NUMBER COMPREHENSION AND COUNTING.** Number comprehension and counting ability may be demonstrated in a child's rote counting, appreciation of number values, and ability to enumerate. These are dependent upon a broad range of functions, most notably:

1. A child must possess adequate auditory, visual, and somatosensory acuity.
2. He must have adequate auditory, visual, and somatosensory discrimination skills.
3. Memory functions must be intact.
4. A child must be able to shift between the visual (e.g., block) and verbal (e.g., number label) modalities.
5. A child's fine motor coordination must be adequate to allow object manipulation and one-to-one counting behavior.
6. He must be able to maintain a one-to-one correspondence between object and number.
7. He must be able to maintain a consistent work pattern.
8. A child must appreciate the association of numbers with quantities as well as with order.

**CALCULATION.** Calculation depends upon a number of ablities including:

1. Number comprehension and counting.
2. Intact sensory acuity and discrimination to allow accurate perception of numbers, function signs (+), and names (addition).
3. Adequate ability to learn verbal-visual (e.g., name-graphic symbol) associations in order to read and write numbers and arithmetic function symbols.
4. Adequate ability to learn associations between specific operations and arithmetic function symbols and the operation procedures themselves.
5. Ablity to learn the number facts.
6. Ability to maintain an appropriate and consistent work pattern.
7. Adequate visual-spatial abilities, which allow a child to maintain the appropriate spatial orientation and organization of written numbers.
8. Adequate ability to remember a sequence of mental manipulations and the operations involved in each.
9. Adequate motor functions for the production of written and oral calculation responses.

**NUMERICAL WORD PROBLEM SOLVING.** This involves the ability to comprehend numbers, count, and calculate. In addition, the ability to solve word problems depends upon basic linguistic and cognitive functions, in particular:

1. Adequate language skills (oral language competence for verbal problems and reading for written ones) to ensure comprehension of the problem at hand and thus to allow translation of the words into numerical operations.
2. Adequate problem solving ability, which involves the ability to visualize the problem as a whole and to plan out and execute the series of operations required to solve it.

## Assessment of Arithmetic and Arithmetic Subskills

Assessment of arithmetic disorders requires the integration of quantitative and qualitative information. Quantitative measures are provided by standardized tests of arithmetic competence and arithmetic subskills. Qualitative information is obtained from many different sources (e.g, reports from parents and schools, special clinical procedures). A summary of representative quantitative and qualitative measures of arithmetic competence and arithmetic subskills is presented in Appendices 15 and 16.

### *Quantitative*

**ARITHMETIC COMPETENCE.** There are standardized tests that variously focus on each of the main aspects of arithmetic competence, namely, number comprehension and counting, calculation, and numerical word problem solving.

**ARITHMETIC SUBSKILLS.** There are standardized tests of subskills such as: visual, auditory, and somatosensory discrimination. There are also standardized tests of grapheme–verbal number associations, visual memory, and auditory memory. Fine motor skills and one-to-one correspondence are assessed quantitatively, as are language functions and general intellectual functions.

### *Qualitative*

The qualitative assessment of a child's arithmetic competence and arithmetic subskills utilizes data obtained from an interview with the parent (or guardian), from school reports, and from clinical observation of the child.

**PARENT (GUARDIAN) REPORT.** Information is obtained about a child's arithmetic skills. A distinction is made between ability to solve word problems mentally and through written calculation. Information is obtained about "practical" number skills (e.g., handling money, telling time) (see Appendix 2).

**SCHOOL REPORT.** The school report provides information about a child's arithmetic competence and subskills (see Appendix 3).

**CLINICAL OBSERVATION.** Clinical observation provides information about the quality of a child's performance: (1) on standardized tests of arithmetic, (2) on age-appropriate numerical tasks, and (3) in spontaneous behavior that involves arithmetic skills. This information is vital to an assessment of arithmetic performance (see Appendix 4).

## REVIEW QUESTIONS

1. Arithmetic disorders are always subordinate to language disturbances. True or False?
2. Arithmetic disorders sometimes involve difficulty organizing numbers into columns. True or False?
3. There are no standardized tests of arithmetic competence. True or False?
4. Name three acquired arithmetic disorder subgroups.
5. Name three characteristics of calculation problems associated with visual-spatial disturbances.
6. In which type of acquired arithmetic disorder is there visual neglect?
7. Which type of arithmetic error pattern is most likely to be associated with right hemisphere dysfunction?
8. What three subskills underlie arithmetic competence?
9. Problems writing numbers in columns and neglect of the left side of visual space are usually associated with dysfuntion in the same brain area. True or False?
10. Describe three errors characteristic of children with an arithmetic disorder.
11. Arithmetic disorders always involve difficulty with enumeration. True or False?

12. Dysgraphia is always associated with dyscalculia. True or False?
13. Reading disorders can cause dyscalculia. True or False?
14. What abilities does the process of enumeration depend on?
15. Describe two abilities underlying the calculation process.

# 12

# EMOTIONAL AND BEHAVIORAL DISORDERS

Parents and teachers are often prompted to seek professional help for a child when they are confronted with emotional and behavioral problems. Among the characteristics of a child with such problems are: moodiness, withdrawal, short attention span, and temper tantrums.

Social, personality, and biological factors, singly and in combination, impact on a child's emotional development and behavior. Each of these influences must be given careful consideration in an assessment of emotional and behavioral disorders in children.

The purpose of this chapter is to offer an overview of the biological determinants of emotional and behavioral disorders. This should in no way imply that: (1) emotional and behavioral disorders are invariably caused by biological disturbance; (2) emotional and behavioral disorders never exist in individuals with normal biological systems; or that (3) individuals with abnormal biological systems always have emotional and behavioral disorders.

In this chapter, we summarize the current understanding of the biological basis of emotion, including a discussion of the reciprocal relation between emotion, behavior, and biological functions; summarize a selected sample of childhood emotional and behavioral disorders; and delineate the diagnostic process.

## BIOLOGICAL BASIS OF EMOTION

Emotion consists of subjective feelings that are accompanied by physiological events. It may also trigger behavior (sometimes referred to as emotional behavior). The biology of emotion is not clearly understood. Current speculation on the

FUNDAMENTALS OF CLINICAL CHILD NEUROPSYCHOLOGY

ISBN 0-8089-1910-5

physiological events in the brain that accompany emotion is based on inferences derived from studies of pathological states in adults and from ablation (removal) and stimulation studies in animals. This body of work suggests that the experience of emotion flows from functional interactions of a number of cortical and subcortical structures and systems. Certain brain chemicals have also been established as having an important role in emotion and emotional behavior.

## Neuroanatomical Basis of Emotion and Emotional Behavior

The neuroanatomical basis of emotion and emotional behavior involves: (1) the frontal lobe, (2) the sensory areas of the cortex, (3) the arousal and selective attention systems, and (4) the limbic system. These have both independent and interactional functions.

### *Frontal Lobe*

The frontal lobe is divided into prefrontal and motor regions. The prefrontal is divided into three regions: (1) the medial, (2) the orbital, and (3) the dorsolateral. The motor is divided into premotor and precentral (motor strip) regions.

The frontal lobe is intimately involved in emotional experience and expression. The region is connected with cortical regions, mainly the association areas. Via the premotor region, the prefrontal area is connected to the precentral cortex. There are also important connections with the limbic and reticular activating systems.

### *Sensory Areas*

The sensory projection areas receive sensory information from the internal and external environment; the sensory association areas interpret the information. An individual's perception and interpretation of this information is used to establish a cognitive set, which is crucial to the experience and expression of emotion.

### *Arousal and Selective Attention System*

The arousal and selective attention system is a functional system that includes the reticular activating system (RAS), the cerebral cortex, and subcortical structures. This system has two crucial roles in the mediation of behavior: (1) it modulates the level of cortical responsiveness to sensory information and (2) it screens incoming sensory information.

Incoming information (except olfactory) reaches the cortex via two pathways. In one the information is sent directly to the cortex; in the other it is sent by way of the reticular activating system.

Sensory information is transmitted through the first (direct) pathway in the following manner. Initially, the stimulus information impinges on a receptor cell. A sensory nerve is activated and a sensory message is transmitted directly through lower brain centers to the primary sensory reception regions. There, the sensory information is further analyzed and interpreted.

In the second (indirect) pathway, sensory information is transmitted to the brain by way of the reticular activating system. This (ascending) pathway transmits excitatory impulses to the entire cortex, affecting both cortical arousal and behavioral arousal.

Feedback pathways between the cortex and many subcortical systems mediate selective attention. The (descending) reticular activating system plays the central role in screening sensory information. The cortex transmits both inhibitory and excitatory instructions back to the (descending) reticular activating system.

Because direct modality specific sensory pathways transmit information to the cortex much more quickly than the indirect pathway (which utilizes ascending RAS fibers), a sensory impulse can reach the cortex through it and send an inhibitory impulse to the RAS before the RAS sends excitatory impulses to the whole cortex. Thus, the modulation of cortical arousal and the filtering of sensory input both occur at the subcortical level and are intimately connected.

### *Limbic System*

The limbic lobe was so designated by Broca in 1878. He called it *"le grand lobe limbique."* As defined today, the limbic system comprises the limbic lobe and certain areas of subcortical and cortical gray matter. It includes parts of the thalamus, hippocampus, amygdala, hypothalamus, mammillary bodies, and certain regions of the frontal and temporal lobes. The structures of the limbic system are organized in complex loops or circuits. (A diagram of the major structures of the limbic system is shown in Figure 12-1.)

The limbic system receives input from a wide range of cortical and subcortical regions. Through its output to cortical and subcortical structures, it mediates a range of behaviors (e.g., feeding, reproduction), some of which have clear emotional components. Within the limbic system, two structures in particular have emerged as having an especially important role in the experience of emotion. These are the thalamus and the hypothalamus.

Certain thalamic nuclei are part of the limbic system. The thalamus is also intimately involved in the activities of the cerebral cortex. Incoming information from the sensory systems is projected to the thalamus and from there is relayed to the cortex. The thalamus serves as a major relay station for all of the senses except olfaction. It also serves as a link between the cerebral cortex and the ascending reticular system.

The hypothalamus is primarily concerned with the maintenance of a relatively constant body environment through the regulation of basic drives, such as thirst and hunger. It is a major connection between the limbic system and the ascending reticular system. Through its input to the autonomic nervous system the hypothalamus mediates the physiological concomitants of emotion. It also affects the endocrine system.

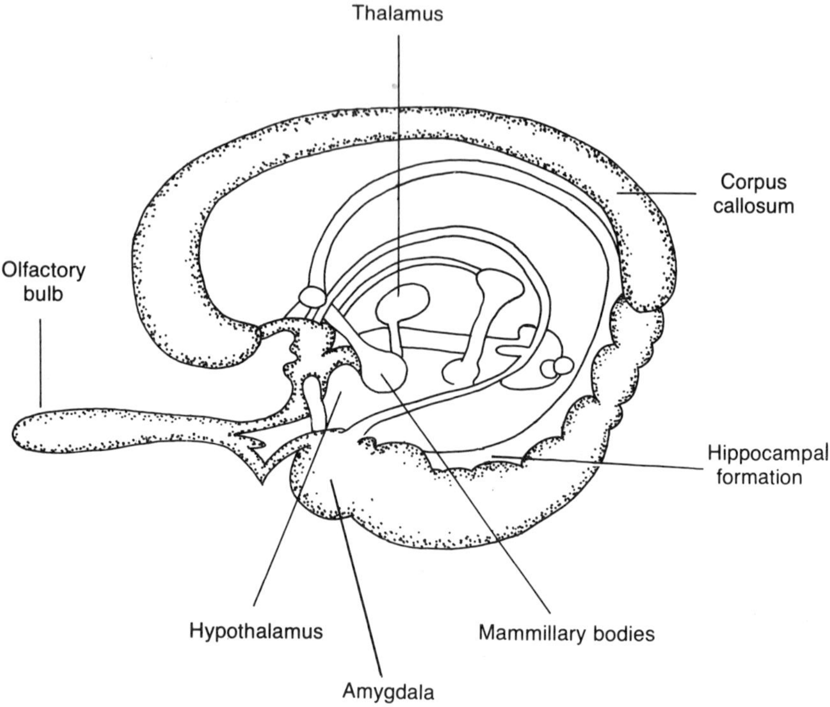


**Figure 12–1.** Major structures of the limbic system. (Adapted with permission from *Clinical Neuropsychology*, 2/e, by K. Heilman and E. Valenstein. Oxford University Press, 1985.)

## Chemical Basis of Emotion and Emotional Behavior

There are three classes of chemicals in the brain that affect neural function and appear to influence emotional states. These are: (1) neurotransmitters, (2) hormones, and (3) neuropeptides. Neurotransmitters are chemicals that are released by presynaptic nerve endings. They may have either excitatory or inhibitory effects on neural impulse transmission. Although any one neuron typically releases only a single neurotransmitter, it may be sensitive to several different neurotranmitters that are released by other neurons. Among the better known neurotransmitters are acetylcholine, the catecholamines (e.g., dopamine and norepinephrine), and serotonin.

Hormones are secreted by the glands and other structures of the endocrine system which is controlled by the hypothalamus. They are released directly into the circulatory system and influence the activities of specific target organs. Glands that are part of the endocrine system include: the pituitary, thyroid, adrenals, pineal body, gonads, and pancreas.

Neuropeptides are a class of chemicals that are produced by some neurons and have stimulating or inhibiting effects on neural activity in the brain. They also have stimulating and inhibiting effects on endocrine and gastrointestinal glands.

## Neuroanatomical Dysfunction and Chemical Imbalance in Emotional and Behavioral Disorders

The effect of biological dysfunction on an individual's emotions and emotional behavior is a topic that has received a great deal of attention. A summary of the relationship between biological condition and emotion and emotional behavior appears in Table 12-1 and is discussed below.

### Neuroanatomical

#### *Frontal Lobe*

The emotional and behavioral consequences of dysfunction in the frontal lobe are associated with the site of dysfunction.

Dysfunction in the mesial aspect of the prefrontal regions is associated with the flattening of affect. Dysfunction in the orbital aspect results in the behavioral characteristics typically associated with the "frontal lobe syndrome." Specifically, while basic intellectual functions remain intact, there is a major disturbance in personality. Features include impulsivity, emotional lability, euphoria, and poor judgement. In contrast, individuals who suffer dysfunction in the dorsolateral region manifest apathetic behavior, psychomotor retardation, motor perseveration, and poor abstraction abilities.

Dysfunction in the frontal motor region of the language dominant hemisphere (usually the left) is associated with disorders in the expression of affect through the production of propositional language. Disorder in the expression of affect through the prosody of speech is associated with dysfunction in the nondominant hemisphere.

#### *Sensory Areas*

Dysfunction of the sensory projection areas is associated with impaired perception and interpretation of information originating in the internal and external environment. This profoundly affects the individual's emotional well-being and adaptive behavior (e.g., a child who fails to interpret voice intonation accurately is likely to have poor social adjustment).

#### *Arousal and Selective Attention System*

The emotional and behavioral effects of dysfunction in the selective arousal and attention system include: indifference, lack of initiative, irritability, distractibility, difficulty concentrating, and difficulty focusing.

#### *Limbic System*

The behavioral effects of limbic system dysfunction in humans and in animals demonstrate the importance of this system in the biology of emotion.

## TABLE 12-1. BIOLOGICAL CONDITIONS ASSOCIATED WITH EMOTION AND EMOTIONAL BEHAVIOR

| BIOLOGICAL CONDITION | EMOTION AND EMOTIONAL BEHAVIOR |
|---|---|
| ***Neuroanatomical*** | |
| ***Frontal Lobe Dysfunction*** | |
| *Mesial* | Flattened affect |
| *Orbitofrontal* | Impulsive behavior<br>Emotional lability<br>Euphoria<br>Poor judgment |
| *Dorsolateral* | Apathetic behavior<br>Psychomotor retardation<br>Motor perseveration<br>Poor abstraction ability |
| *Motor* | Disorder in expression of affect through production of propositional language (dominant hemisphere)<br>Difficulty in expression of affect through prosody (nondominant hemisphere) |
| ***Sensory Area Dysfunction*** | Inappropriate emotional responses<br>Maladaptive behavior |
| ***Arousal and Selective Attention System Dysfunction*** | Lack of initiative<br>Irritability<br>Distractibility<br>Difficulty concentrating<br>Difficulty focusing |
| ***Limbic System Dysfunction*** | Placidity<br>Rage-like behavior<br>Impulsivity<br>Depression<br>Schizophrenia (Type 2)<br>Emotional features of complex partial seizures |
| ***Lateralized Cortical Dysfunction*** | |
| *Right hemisphere* | Difficulty interpreting and expressing affect through prosody and visual cues<br>Lack of awareness of effect of behavior on others<br>Failure to recognize own condition |
| *Left hemisphere* | Difficulty understanding and expressing affect through propositional language<br>"Catastrophic reaction"<br>Indifference reaction<br>Flattened affect |
| ***Chemical*** | |
| *Chemical imbalance* | Schizophrenia (Type 1)<br>Manic-depressive disorder<br>Depression<br>Premenstrual disorder<br>Aggressive behavior<br>Secondary psychosis<br>Sexual hypo/hyperarousal<br>"Runner's high" |

**HUMAN STUDIES.** Studies of diseases affecting the limbic system have suggested that bilateral temporal lobe lesions involving limbic structures produce placidity; that tumors in a focal region produce rage and irritability (whereas stimulation of the same region produces intense pleasure). It has also been reported that diseases such as herpes simplex encephalitis, which affect the limbic system, result in behavioral abnormalities, including impulsivity and depression, as well as in memory loss. Subcortical dysfunction has also been implicated in some affective disorders. For example, the importance of hypothalamic dysfunction in certain violent patients has been suggested by the success of hypothalamotomy in their treatment.

Acquired dysfunction of the limbic or limbic-related regions has been associated with one subtype of schizophrenia.

Certain epileptic seizure disorders have specific emotional features. Emotional symptomology tends to occur particularly in complex partial seizures when the focus of the epileptic seizure is in a region of the temporal lobe which is in or near the limbic system. The emotional phenomena are divided into: (1) ictal, (2) postictal, and (3) interictal. Ictal (during seizure) phenomena include affective automatisms (laughing and crying) and strong emotions (e.g., anxiety). Postictal (after seizure) phenomena include confusion and restlessness. A controversial body of literature suggests that individuals who have complex partial seizures may also experience interictal (between seizure) changes in personality, including such features as anxiety and depression. The possible existence of a distinct personality pattern (e.g., hyperreligiosity, interest in the abstract) has also been discussed.

**ANIMAL STUDIES.** Stimulation and ablation (removal) techniques have been used to study the role of the limbic system. Although there are theoretical and methodological difficulties in extrapolating from this body of research to humans, important findings have nevertheless emerged. In fact, a number of the findings are analogous to those obtained in studies of human patients. For example:

Bilateral removal of the anterior temporal lobe results in a behavior pattern known as the Kluver-Bucy syndrome. This syndrome, which was first observed in monkeys (and is also seen in humans), is characterized by a dramatic change in behavior in which an aggressive and wild animal becomes tame, docile, and hyposexual. Lesions in certain other parts of the limbic system produce rage-like behavior.

### *Lateralized Dysfunction*

Dysfunction of the right side of the cerebral cortex in adults may result in difficulty in the interpretation and expression of affect through the prosody of speech. An individual suffering from right hemispheric dysfunction has difficulty understanding and expressing emotion via visual cues, such as facial expression and gestures. Additionally, he often tends to be oblivious to the effect of his behavior on others and is unaware of his own condition.

By contrast, an individual with left (usually dominant) hemisphere dysfunction has difficulty understanding or expressing emotion on the basis of propositional language.

**TABLE 12-2. REPRESENTATIVE CHARACTERISTICS AND POSTULATED ETIOLOGY OF TWO SCHIZOPHRENIA SUBTYPES**

| |
|---|
| **TYPE 1** |
| ***"Positive" Symptoms*** |
| Hallucinations |
| Thought disorder |
| Delusions |
| ***Postulated Etiology*** |
| Inherited disorder of dopamine metabolism |
| Inherited disorder of dopamine receptor sensitivity |
| **TYPE 2** |
| ***"Negative" Symptoms*** |
| Social withdrawal |
| Flattened affect |
| ***Postulated Etiology*** |
| Acquired dysfunction of limbic or limbic-related regions |

He may be able to convey emotion through prosody. He may experience "catastrophic reaction" (i.e., profound depression), indifference reaction, or flattened affect.

## Chemical

### *Neurotransmitters*

Two subtypes of schizophrenia have been identified: Type 1 and Type 2. Type 1 is characterized by "positive symptoms," e.g., hallucinations, thought disorder, delusions. Type 2 is characterized by "negative symptoms," e.g., social withdrawal, flattened affect. Type 1 schizophrenia appears to be associated with inherited disorders of dopamine metabolism or in dopamine receptor sensitivity, whereas Type 2 is thought to result from an acquired dysfunction of limbic or limbic-related areas. Characteristics of the two subtypes of schizophrenia are summarized in Table 12–2.

The symptoms of manic-depressive and certain other depressive illnesses have also been attributed to fluctuations in neurotransmitter levels in critical areas of the brain.

The therapeutic effects of psychotropic medication are thought to be consequences of their restorative effect on the concentrations of particular neurotransmitters.

### *Hormones*

Endocrine alteration has been associated with: (1) premenstrual disorders, (2) depression, (3) aggressive and violent behavior, and (4) secondary psychosis (e.g., postpartum psychosis).

### *Neuropeptides*

Neuropeptides serve as inhibitory or excitatory influences. Among the behaviors they affect are sexual behavior.

Endorphins are a class of neuropeptides found in the brain that have received a great deal of attention in the psychology research literature. They are released when an individual is under stress and function as natural painkillers. The "runner's high" is considered an example of the consequences of increased release of endorphins.

Animal research indicates that a decreased level of endorphins results in an increased sensitivity to pain.

## EMOTIONAL AND BEHAVIORAL DISORDERS IN CHILDREN

Emotional and behavioral disorders can be divided into two groups: organic and nonorganic. An organic mental disorder is a constellation of emotional and behavioral symptoms associated with either known or presumed, permanent or transient, specific brain dysfunction that is etiologically associated with the abnormal mental condition. A nonorganic mental disorder is a constellation of emotional and behavioral symptoms that is traditionally accounted for by psychological, social, and/or familial interpersonal factors.

In this section we discuss a selected sample of nonorganic emotional and behavioral disorders in children. We describe the essential features of the disorders and note current biological research findings (seen in the adult and child literature) that point to the presence of organic factors in a number of these disorders.

The major nonorganic emotional and behavioral disorders in children can be classified as (1) developmental disorders, (2) emotional disorders, and (3) disruptive behavioral disorders. The first group includes pervasive developmental disorder and infantile autism. The second group includes anxiety disorders, mood disorders, adjustment disorder, personality disorders, and schizophrenia. The third group includes attention-deficit hyperactivity disorder and conduct disorder. Table 12–3 summarizes selected emotional and behavioral disorders in children.

### Developmental Disorders

#### *Pervasive Developmental Disorder*

A pervasive developmental disorder is characterized by a serious distortion in the development of basic psychological functions. In contrast to the specific developmental disorders (of reading, writing, and arithmetic), a pervasive developmental disorder involves multiple areas of development. It is characterized

**TABLE 12-3. EMOTIONAL AND BEHAVIORAL DISORDERS IN CHILDREN**

I. Developmental disorders
   A. Pervasive developmental disorder
   B. Infantile autism
II. Emotional disorders
   A. Anxiety disorders
   B. Mood disorders
   C. Adjustment Disorder
   D. Personality disorders
   E. Schizophrenia
III. Disruptive behavioral disorders
   A. Attention-deficit hyperactivity disorder
   B. Conduct disorder

primarily by: profound disruption of verbal and nonverbal communication, markedly poor social interaction, and impaired symbolic behavior.

The biological basis of pervasive developmental disorder is poorly understood. The symptoms suggest, however, that both cortical and subcortical functions are impaired.

### *Infantile Autism*

Infantile autism is a severe form of pervasive developmental disorder. It may be associated with deficited intellectual skills, abnormal postures and movements, atypical sleeping and eating habits.

The biological basis of infantile autism is not well understood. The profound and pervasive nature of the symptomology in this disorder suggest that diffuse brain dysfunction is involved.

## Emotional Disorders

### *Anxiety Disorders*

Anxiety, or feelings of apprehension in the absence of manifest danger, is the major symptom of this group of disorders. Anxiety disorders are characterized by persistent excessive or unrealistic worry. Somatic components are common. Currently, anxiety disorders are subdivided on the basis of whether the anxiety is triggered by a specific situation or a variety of situations.

Biological models of anxiety disorders typically attribute the symptomology to excessive activity of the subcortical systems.

### *Mood Disorders*

This group of disorders is characterized by disturbances of mood. Symptoms of depression or of elation may predominate. Mood disorders are commonly divided into bipolar and depressive subgroups. The bipolar group is characterized by depression and mania. The depressive is characterized by depression. The essential features of a manic episode is an elated, expansive, or irritable mood with specific associated symptoms, such as inflated self-esteem, decreased need for sleep, and psychomotor agitation. A depressive episode is characterized by a depressed or an irritable mood or loss of interest or pleasure in usual activities. Associated symptoms include psychomotor agitation or retardation, sleep and eating disturbances.

Mood disorders in children are most frequently of the depressive type.

Dysfunction of the limbic system and other subcortical structures has been associated with mood disorders. Abnormalities involving the neurotransmitter norepinephrine have also been suggested.

### *Adjustment Disorder*

The essential feature of an adjustment disorder is a maladaptive reaction to a psychostressor, or stressors (e.g., parental death). It is assumed that the maladaptive behavior will stop when the stressor ceases or when new adaptive skills develop. The maladaptive reaction is manifested as either extreme reactions to the stressor (e.g., marked social withdrawal) or impairment in (school) functioning.

The adjustment disorder is subdivided on the basis of presenting clinical picture.

There is currently no clear evidence suggesting that an adjustment disorder is associated with organic factors.

### *Personality Disorders*

The personality disorder subgroup of emotional disorders in children is controversial.

A personality disorder is one in which an individual's personality traits are inflexible and impede his adaptive functioning, socially and academically. This inflexibility is often experienced as distressful. Associated features of personality disorders are mood disturbances.

Personality disorders are divided into subgroups on the basis of predominant adaptive style.

The majority of the personality disorder types have not been associated with organic dysfunction. However, there are suggestions of underlying biological disturbances in some personality disorder subtypes (e.g., borderline).

### *Schizophrenia*

This disorder is characterized by psychotic behavior and by deterioration of a previously attained level of functioning. The disorder typically involves disturbances in perception, affect, self-image, volition, thinking, and psychomotor behavior.

Schizophrenia is often considered to be the consequence of internal and external factors acting in concert. An individual predisposed to the illness by internal factors is more vulnerable than others to particular environmental factors, which serve to trigger or to induce a psychotic episode. Research suggests that internal precipitating factors include inherited disorder of neurotransmitter metabolism or receptor sensitivity and acquired dysfunction in limbic or limbic-related areas.

### Disruptive Behavioral Disorders

#### *Attention-Deficit Hyperactivity Disorder*

Over the years, a combination of behaviors, seen in the classroom and at home, has been given many labels, including: minimal brain damage and minimal brain dysfunction (MBD), hyperkinesis syndrome, hyperactive child syndrome, and attention deficit disorder with (ADD-H) and without (ADD) hyperactivity. Today, attention-deficit hyperactivity disorder (A-DHD) is the accepted diagnostic label.

The basic features of an attention-deficit hyperactivity disorder (A-DHD) are a degree and frequency of restlessness and difficulty paying attention that are more excessive than expected for an individual of a given mental age. Associated features of this disorder are fidgetiness, distractiblity, impulsivity, difficulty awaiting one's turn, difficulty following directions and completing activities, and poor ability to organize.

In mild cases, the attention-deficit hyperactivity disorder is associated with little or no impairment in functioning at school or with peers. In severe cases, there is pervasive and serious impairment in functioning at school, socially, and at home.

Investigators have suggested that attention-deficit hyperactivity disorder is the consequence of dysfunction in the complex subcortical and cortical brain structures and pathways that underlie arousal and selective attention. The primary structures involved in arousal and selective attention are the: (1) cerebral cortex, (2) thalamus, (3) reticular activating system (RAS), and (4) the limbic system.

#### *Conduct Disorder*

The basic feature of a conduct disorder is a persistent and repetitive conduct pattern in which age-appropriate social rules are seriously violated. The disorder is typically manifested in a variety of settings and often involves physical aggression. This disorder is commonly associated with poor frustration tolerance, poor academic achievement, poor self-esteem, and symptoms of anxiety and depression.

Although biological dysfunction has not been associated with conduct disorder, its associated features strongly suggest that organic dysfunction is likely to exist.

## DIAGNOSIS OF EMOTIONAL AND BEHAVIORAL DISORDERS

The diagnosis of emotional and behavioral disorders is an extremely complex and challenging task. Diagnostic tools today permit only a limited assessment of the contributions of social, personality, and biological factors to these disorders. At no point should the psychologist assume that dramatic evidence pointing to personality factors necessarily precludes the existence of biological factors. Similarly, he should never assume that clear biological factors preclude the existence of important personality contributions. In the vast majority of cases, the psychologist who recognizes the existence of an emotional or behavioral disorder in a child is likely to be dealing with the interaction of multiple factors.

The diagnosis of emotional and behavioral disorders requires the integration of quantitative and qualitative information. Qualititative information is obtained from a variety of sources (e.g., reports from parent (guardian) and school, clinical observation).

### *Quantitative*

There are a number of formal measures of personality and of emotional status. Grouped under the general heading of projective techniques, these assessment tools also allow the trained psychologist to obtain a sense of a child's emotional strengths and weaknesses and areas of conflict.

### *Qualitative*

**PARENT (GUARDIAN) REPORT.** The psychologist asks the parent (or guardian) for a detailed description of the presenting condition. He also obtains information regarding possible precipitating factors and factors that serve to exacerbate or ameliorate the problem behavior.

A complete history must be obtained. The history of emotional and behavioral development must include the age of onset of disturbances and the occurrence of any traumata that might affect development. Information regarding medical and family background is crucial (see Appendix 2).

**SCHOOL REPORT.** The school report supplies information regarding a child's emotional development and behavior, as well as his academic performance (Appendix 3).

**CLINICAL OBSERVATION.** In formulating an overall clinical impression of the child, the psychologist should carefully observe the child's physical appearance and behavior. A child's motor activity level and apparent emotional state should also be noted.

Tests of cognitive and intellectual abilities are not considered measures of emotion and emotional behavior, but they may provide important information in this regard. During administration of these tests, the psychologist notes such patterns as personal reference, intratest and intertest variability (see Appendix 4).

## REVIEW QUESTIONS

1. MBD and A-DHD refer to distinctive behavioral syndromes. True or False?
2. Name two important neuroanatomical systems that have important functions in emotion and emotional behavior.
3. The frontal lobe is most crucial in emotion and emotional behavior. True or False?
4. Within the limbic system, which two structures have an especially important role in emotion and emotional behavior?
5. What two classes of brain chemicals are important in emotion and emotional behavior?
6. Describe the effects on emotion and emotional behavior of dysfunction in the right cerebral hemisphere.
7. Describe the effects on emotion and emotional behavior of dysfunction in the prefrontal lobes.
8. What is the "frontal lobe syndrome"?
9. What are the effects of stimulation of the limbic system?
10. Describe the Kluver-Bucy syndrome.
11. Describe two subtypes of schizophrenia.
12. What are some effects of neuropeptide imbalance?
13. Name the major classes of emotional and behavioral disorders in children.
14. Name two developmental disorders of childhood.
15. Define organic and nonorganic mental disorders.

# 13

# COMPREHENSIVE PSYCHOLOGICAL EVALUATION

Learning problems, emotional disorders, and behavior problems are symptoms of underlying disturbances. The underlying disturbances may be social, emotional, and/or biological in nature. It is only through a comprehensive assessment of each of these factors that a psychologist is able to:

1. Determine a child's level of functioning and areas of strength and weakness
2. Diagnose the underlying dysfunctions and define their interrelationships
3. Develop effective treatment strategies

In this chapter, we give an overview of a comprehensive psychological evaluation and summarize the typical recommendations and treatment strategies.

## COMPREHENSIVE PSYCHOLOGICAL EVALUATION

In our view, a comprehensive psychological evaluation must assess the social, emotional, and neuropsychological (brain-behavior) factors that singly or in combination impact on a child's growth and development. The components of such an examination are summarized in Table 13–1.

### Social

The social factors that impact on a child's learning, emotional well-being, and be-

FUNDAMENTALS OF CLINICAL CHILD NEUROPSYCHOLOGY


ISBN 0-8089-1910-5

**TABLE 13-1. COMPREHENSIVE PSYCHOLOGICAL EVALUATION**

| |
|---|
| HISTORY |
| SCHOOL REPORT |
| CLINICAL OBSERVATION |
| PERSONALITY ASSESSMENT |
| INTELLIGENCE ASSESSMENT |
| SPEECH ASSESSMENT |
| LANGUAGE ASSESSMENT |
| *Competence* |
| *Subskills* |
| ACADEMIC SKILLS ASSESSMENT |
| *Competence* |
| *Subskills* |
| SELECTED NEUROPSYCHOLOGICAL FUNCTION ASSESSMENT |
| OTHER SPECIALIZED EVALUATION PROCEDURES AS NEEDED: |
| *Neurological* |
| *Psychiatric* |
| *Ophthalmological* |
| *Audiological* |
| *Speech/Language* |

havior are defined by his family and his community. The psychologist makes an assessment of these social factors based on the integration of information obtained through (1) interview of the child's parent (or guardian), (2) school report, (3) interview with and observation of the child, and (4) the psychologist's general knowledge of the child's culture and community.

The evaluation begins with an interview of the child's parent (or guardian). In addition to information regarding the presenting problem(s), the psychologist obtains data on the child's developmental, medical, social, and academic histories. A concise yet complete family history is gathered. A general outline of the information to be obtained is presented in Appendix 2. A school report is also obtained (Appendix 3). The educational philosophy of the child's school regarding academics and discipline is also important information to be noted.

The child is also asked about his personal and family histories. His impressions of his school and his neighborhood are noted. Observation of his appearance and his style of interaction as they may impact on his social adaptation are also noted (Appendix 4).

It is incumbent upon the psychologist to familiarize himself as much as possible with the general character of the culture and community in which a child is being raised.

## Emotional

A child's emotional well-being and personality structure impact profoundly on his ability to learn and to function adaptively and effectively. A child's emotional status and personality are assessed through: (1) the description of a child offered by the parent (or guardian), (2) school report, (3) interpretation of the child's performance on standardized measures, and (4) clinical observations.

During the initial meeting with the parent (or guardian), the psychologist obtains a general description of the child, in terms of traits, interests, and style of functioning at home, in school, and in the community. A school report is also obtained.

Performance on two different types of tests must be carefully evaluated: (1) formal tests of personality structure and functions and (2) tests of cognitive and intellectual abilities. Through interpretation of the child's performance on these assessment tools, it is possible for the trained professional to define many aspects of personality (e.g., areas of conflict, ego strength, defense style).

The standard measures of personality (also called projective techniques) that are frequently used are:

1. Rorschach technique. The Rorschach consists of ten symmetrical inkblots printed on a white background. Five of the inkblots are varying shades of gray; two are red and gray; three are multicolored. The child is presented with the plates one at a time and is asked to tell the examiner what the blots look like. An inquiry to gain clearer understanding of the response follows.

2. Thematic Apperception Test (TAT). The TAT consists of a total of thirty pictures, representing people of both sexes at different ages, depicted alone and in groups, in various settings, and in various types of interactions. The usual number of cards shown is ten.

The child is presented with the pictures one at a time and asked to tell a spontaneous story about the people depicted.

3. Children's Apperception Test (CAT). The CAT consists of a series of ten pictures depicting dressed animal figures in various human settings and situations. The CAT was designed to be used with younger children. The child is presented with the pictures one at a time and asked to tell a spontaneous story about the figures depicted. The CAT-H is a version of the CAT in which the animal figures are changed to human figures.

4. House-Tree-Person Test (H-T-P). The H-T-P is a projective drawing test. It consists of a series of four spontaneous drawings. The child is asked to sketch without a model a house, a tree, and a person. A second human figure of the sex opposite to the one initially drawn is also requested.

During administration of tests of cognitive and intellectual functioning, the psychologist notes the individual's performance (e.g., idyosyncratic responses and intratest and intertest response variability).

While working with the child, the psychologist forms a clinical impression, based on the child's appearance, behavior, and verbalizations. The child is assessed descriptively, as well as in terms of the appropriateness of his presentation for his age and sex. A general outline of the information used to form a clinical impression is presented in Appendix 4.

### Neuropsychological

Biological dysfunction of the brain is manifested by perceptual and sensory disorders, deficits in motor functions, defects in cognitive skills and specific learning skills, impaired speech/language functions, and epileptic seizure phenomena. Emotional and behavioral disorders may also reflect underlying biological dysfunction. A subtle biological dysfunction can have a profound impact on a child's intellectual growth, emotional well-being, and social development.

The evaluation of neuropsychological factors requires the integration of a broad range of information. From an interview with the child's parent (or guardian), the psychologist obtains data on the child's (1) pre-, peri-, and postnatal histories, (2) developmental milestones, (3) medical history, (4) social history, (5) academic history, and (6) family history. A school report is also obtained.

During meetings with the child, the psychologist assesses his neuropsychological functioning through both quantitative and qualitative measures. The quantitative measures are standardized tests. The psychologist assesses the following areas:

1. Intelligence
2. Speech
3. Language competence and language subskills
4. Academic competence and academic subskills
5. Selected neuropsychological functions

The qualitative measures include those obtained by:

1. Noting the quality of the child's performance on standardized tests
2. Asking the child to perform age-appropriate tasks
3. Noting the child's spontaneous behavior and verbalizations

Table 13-2 presents representative neuropsychological functions assessed in a comprehensive psychological evaluation.

## RECOMMENDATIONS

Based on the results of the evaluation, the psychologist makes recommendations for: (1) further evaluations and/or (2) prescriptive treatment.

### Further Evaluations

Not infrequently, after completing the comprehensive psychological evaluation, the psychologist recommends ancillary evaluations. These evaluations are recommended in order to: (1) establish a medical diagnosis or (2) more clearly delineate a diagnosed disorder. Among the referrals most frequently made are those to a specialist in neurology, psychiatry, ophthalmology, audiology, and speech/language pathology.

**TABLE 13-2. REPRESENTATIVE* NEUROPSYCHOLOGICAL FUNCTIONS ASSESSED IN A COMPREHENSIVE PSYCHOLOGICAL EVALUATION**

I. Sensory Acuity and Perceptual Discrimination
   A. Auditory
   B. Visual
   C. Somatosensory
II. Motor Functions
   A. Fine
   B. Gross
   C. Ocular
   D. Integrative
      1. Graphomotor
      2. Dyspraxia
III. Memory
   A. Auditory
   B. Visual
   C. Somatosensory
IV. Touch and Body Schema
   A. Tactile Recognition
   B. Finger Recognition
   C. Right-Left Orientation
V. Dominance
   A. Hand
   B. Foot
   C. Eye
VI. Space
   A. Work Pattern
   B. Spatial Orientation
   C. Spatial Organization
VII. Time
VIII. Speech
IX. Language
   A. Automatic
   B. Receptive
   C. Expressive

*The neuropsychological functions outlined in the above table are not inclusive. They are meant to serve as a guide in the development of an evaluation procedure to be modified as needed, in individual cases, by the psychologist.

**NEUROLOGY.** A child is referred to a neurologist if his history, performance on tests, behavior and/or verbalizations show evidence of: (1) epileptic seizure disorder, (2) significant sensory or motor disorder, (3) attention deficit-hyperactivity disorder, or under special circumstances, (4) headaches.

Laboratory tests are commonly recommended by the neurologist. The decision to order laboratory tests and the types of tests ordered are based on the child's history and the findings of the neurological examination. Among those most frequently used are:

1. Electroencephalogram (EEG). This test yields information on the electrophysiological activity of the brain. It is central to the diagnosis of epileptic seizure disorders.

2. Computerized transaxial tomography (CT scan). This is an x-ray procedure that produces images of the brain's structure. It is used to reveal tumors, blood clots, and other structural abnormalities.

**PSYCHIATRY.** A referral to a psychiatrist is made when data from a child's history, test performance, and/or behavior and verbalizations suggest the possible utility of drug therapy or the value of a consultation regarding diagnosis.

**OPHTHAMOLOGY.** A child is referred to an ophthalmologist when his history, test performance, and/or behavior and verbalizations suggest: (1) diminished visual acuity, (2) impaired ocular motility, or (3) visual field defects.

**AUDIOLOGY.** Because hearing defects frequently masquerade as poor language or speech development, and vice versa, a referral is made to an audiologist whenever a child's history, test performance, and/or behavior and verbalizations suggest: (1) language dysfunction, (2) speech disorder, or (3) diminished hearing acuity.

**SPEECH/LANGUAGE PATHOLOGY.** A child whose history, performance on tests, or clinical presentation suggest a significant speech/language disorder is referred to a specialist in speech/language pathology for further evaluation.

## Prescriptive Treatment

Given a determination of level of functioning, strengths and weaknesses, and a diagnosis of underlying dysfunctions, the goal of follow-up treatment is to facilitate a child's growth and development. To accomplish this goal, a variety of intervention modalities may be utilized, singly or in combination. The strategies may include: (1) remediation, (2) psychotherapy, (3) counseling, and (4) medication.

# GLOSSARY

**Afferent neural pathways:** transmit impulses from the body toward or into the central nervous system.

**Agnosia:** the inability to recognize a familiar stimulus or class of stimuli despite intact sensory processes. Agnosia is usually specific for a particular sensory system and for a subcategory of stimuli within that system (e.g., nonspeech sounds, speech sounds, colors, visually presented objects).

**Agraphesthesia:** a somatosensory disorder characterized by inability to recognize a shape, number, or letter that is "written" on the hand.

**Amnesia:** a severe memory deficit that impairs long-term memory. Short-term memory, level of general intellectual functioning.

**Amygdala:** a structure in the limbic system.

**Angular gyrus:** located at the temporal-parietal junction, adjacent to the occipital lobe. The dominant angular gyrus is thought to have a central role in cortical functions such as reading.

**Anterograde amnesia:** the inability to learn new material. Individuals with this type of disturbance tend to be disoriented and may also confabulate.

**Aphasia:** an acquired language disturbance that involves impairment (or loss) of normal language resulting from a dysfunction of the brain that occurs after language has developed.

**Astereognosis:** the inability to recognize an object by palpatation on the basis of its three-dimensionality.

**Auditory agnosia:** the inability to recognize familiar nonspeech and speech sounds in the presence of normal hearing.

**Auditory cortex:** the region of the temporal lobe that receives and interprets auditory information.

**Auditory discrimination disorder:** the inability to discriminate sounds. In fairly mild cases, it may involve only sounds ( nonspeech or speech) that are very much alike. In severe cases, it involves inability to discriminate any nonspeech or speech sounds.

**Aura:** the symptom of a focal seizure (e.g., an auditory hallucination). It is experienced prior to a secondarily generalized epileptic seizure.

**Autonomic nervous system:** functions automatically and reflexively, having a large degree of independence from the central nervous system. It sends commands to the glands and smooth muscles of the skin, the visceral organs, and the blood vessels. It has two divisions, the parasympathetic and the sympathetic.

**Axon:** a subdivision of a neuron. It transmits neural impulses to other cells and to effector organs.

**Babinski reflex:** obtained by stroking the side of the foot from the heel crossing to the big toe, with a pointed object. The normal response is flexion of all toes or no response. The abnormal response is dorsiflexion of the big toe and fanning of the other toes.

**Basal ganglia:** masses of gray matter in the interior cerebrum. They are part of the extrapyramidal (motor) system. Dysfunction results in motor disturbances, including rigidity and resting tremors.

**Body schema (body image):** an individual's spatial perception of his own body.

**Brain:** consists of the: (1) cerebrum, (2) deep structures, (3) cerebellum, and (4) brain stem. The brain and spinal cord make up the central nervous system. The deep structures include the diencephalon, the basal ganglia, and structures of the limbic system.

**Brain dysfunction:** a term that may refer to structural, chemical, and/or biochemical abnormalities that occur in the brain or to the consequences of such abnormalities on brain functions (e.g., motor disorders, seizure disorders, language disorders).

**Brain stem:** a structure that lies between the inner core of the cerebrum and the spinal cord. It comprises the midbrain, pons, and medulla.

**Broca's (motor) aphasia:** an expressive aphasia characterized by a paucity of spontaneous speech with preserved comprehension and impaired naming and repetition ability.

**Broca's area:** located in the dominant, usually left, inferior frontal gyrus. It is responsible for the verbal encoding of language.

**Brodmann's system:** delineates regions of the brain based on cellular structure, yielding a cytoarchitectural "map" of the cortex.

**Central nervous system (CNS):** made up of the brain and spinal cord.

**Cerebellum:** a large structure at the base of the cerebrum. It controls equilibrium, muscle tone, and motor coordination. Cerebellar dysfunction is reflected in motor signs that are ipsilateral to the dysfunction site.

**Cerebral cortex:** the outer layer of the cerebrum. It is gray in color and comprised of densely packed and intricately interconnected, unmyelinated nerve tracts. The cortex is deeply folded and convoluted.

**Cerebral lateralization:** refers to asymmetry of function between the right and left cerebral hemispheres.

**Cerebrum:** comprises two cerebral hemispheres. The cerebral hemispheres are divided into regions on the basis of structure and function. The four major regions are the occipital, temporal, parietal, and frontal lobes.

**Circumlocutions:** convoluted ways of saying things, commonly used by individuals with word finding problems who tend to substitute words in situations where they cannot come up with the word they need.

**Complex partial seizures (temporal lobe seizures and psychomotor seizures):** epileptic seizures in which consciousness is always affected to some degree. Psychic, autonomic, psychosensory, and psychomotor disturbances may occur.

**Computerized transaxial tomography (CT scan):** a powerful radiological technique that provides three-dimensional images of the brain. It is used to reveal tumors, blood clots, and other structural abnormalities.

**Conduction aphasia:** a mixed receptive-expressive aphasia. It is primarily characterized by a severe disturbance in the ability to repeat words despite normal comprehension of oral language and relatively intact fluency.

**Conductive (or transmission) deafness:** diminished sensitivity to sound as a result of dysfunction of the outer or middle ear.

**Contralateral:** opposite side. It is commonly used in describing the relationship in which one side of the cerebral cortex controls the sensory and motor functions on the opposite side of the body.

**Corpus callosum:** the largest commissure. It connects the majority of the cortical regions of the right and left cerebral hemispheres and provides the pathways necessary for communication between the hemispheres.

**Cranial nerves:** transmit impulses from and to the head, the neck region, and some visceral areas. They are part of the peripheral nervous system.

**Critical periods:** commonly defined as periods of rapid neurobiological development, anatomical or functional, during which the organism is maximally sensitive to certain specific as well as other nonspecific external stimuli.

**CT scan:** see computerized transaxial tomography.

**Dendrite:** a subdivision of a neuron. Typically, it has many branches. It receives information from sensory receptors or other neurons.

**Diencephalon:** deep region of the brain that includes such structures as the thalamus, hypothalamus, pituitary gland, pineal gland, and mammillary bodies.

**Dominant:** a term typically used to describe a hand preference or to describe the cerebral hemisphere (usually the left) that is responsible for language functions.

**Dyscalculia:** a developmental arithmetic disorder that is characterized by the failure to develop arithmetic competence.

**Dysgraphia:**a developmental writing disorder that is characterized by the failure to develop writing competence.

**Dyslexia:** a developmental reading disorder that is characterized by the failure to develop reading competence.

**Dysorthographia:** a term used to refer to all cases (acquired and developmental) of written spelling disturbance.

**Dysphasia:** a developmental language disturbance that involves failure to develop language or delayed or deviant acquisition of language.

**Dyspraxia:** a disturbance in the ability to execute a previously learned motor skill accurately upon verbal command.

**Echolalia:** a language disturbance in which the individual repeats the word(s) spoken to him.

**Efferent neural pathways:** transmit neural impulses from the central nervous system to effector organs.

**Electroencephalogram (EEG):** a record of the alternating excitatory and inhibitory electrical activity of the neurons in the brain. The record is obtained by placing a set of electrodes on the scalp in a special arrangement.

**Epilepsy:** a condition characterized by recurrent epileptic seizures.

**Epileptic seizures:** the result of paroxysmal alterations in neuronal activity in the brain. The discharges are abnormal and uncontrolled. They are variously manifested in episodes of disturbance of consciousness, language, cognition, affect, sensory experience, and behavior.

**Episodic memory:** a form of long-term memory that refers to an individual's memory for events in his own life.

**Extrapyramidal system:** one of the two motor systems that control human motor activity. It mediates alterations in body posture and coordination of voluntary movements that are initiated by the pyramidal system.

**Febrile seizures:** a type of infant and childhood seizure. They are usually generalized and of a short duration. They occur soon after the onset of a fever or at the peak of a fever.

**Finger agnosia:** the inability to recognize or identify one's own individual fingers or those of someone else.

**Frontal lobe:** a main division of the cerebral cortex. It is responsible for the highest level of integration of information and for motor activities.

**Generic memory:** a form of long-term memory that refers to an individual's memory for items of general knowledge. It represents the sum total of all that an individual has learned.

**Gerstmann syndrome:** a syndrome characterized by four disturbances: (1) finger agnosia, (2) right-left disorientation, (3) writing disorder, and (4) arithmetic disorder. This syndrome is often associated with language and constructional disturbances.

**Gilles de la Tourette's syndrome:** a neurological syndrome involving abnormal involuntary movements in which children develop verbal tics (usually seen as involuntary cursing) as well as multiple motor tics.

**Glial cells (neuroglia):** cells in the nervous system that are not neurons. They have structural and nutritional roles.

**Golgi type I:** a type of neuron that represents the majority of neurons in the nervous system. It is usually large, with long axons and multiply branched dendrites.

**Golgi type II:** a type of neuron found in the nervous system that is usually small and is thought to be important for higher cerebral functions.

**Grand mal seizures:** generalized epileptic seizures, also referred to as tonic-clonic seizures. In these epileptic seizures, consciousness is always lost. There is also violent motor activity. The motor activity has two phases: first the tonic, then the clonic.

**Gray matter:** those nervous system regions composed of densely packed and intricately interconnected unmyelinated fibers. They are called gray matter because of their gray color.

**Handedness:** defined as either hand preference or as a difference between hands in skill level. Approximately 90% of all people are right-handed. The rest are either left-handed or ambidextrous.

**Haptic imperception:** the inability to recognize the texture, size, and shape of an object through exploration with the hand.

**Hippocampus:** a structure in the limbic system that plays an important role in memory functions.

**Hypertonia:** a muscle tone disturbance characterized by increased muscle tone. It is manifested by an increase in the resistance of a person's limb when it is passively moved through the range of motion.

**Hypothalamus:** a subcortical structure in the central nervous system. It is part of the limbic system and is involved in many crucial emotional and basic physiological functions.

**Hypotonia:** a muscle tone disturbance characterized by decreased muscle tone. It is manifested by a decrease in the resistance of an individual's limb when it is moved passively through the range of motion.

**Ideational dyspraxia:** a type of dyspraxia that is reflected in a difficulty performing upon verbal command previously learned complex motor acts that can be performed spontaneously, for example, pouring and drinking a glass of milk.

**Ideomotor dyspraxia:** a type of dyspraxia that is reflected in a difficulty performing upon verbal command a previously learned simple motor act that can be performed spontaneously, for example, waving good-bye.

**Intention tremors:** tremors that are prominent during movement and become more pronounced during the performance of a task.

**Interictal period:** the period of time between epileptic seizures.

**Intraictal period:** the period of time during an epileptic seizure.

**Ipsilateral:** same side. It is commonly used in describing the relationship in which one side of the brain controls the sensory and motor functions on the same side of the body.

**Jacksonian march:** one phase of a partial seizure with motor symptoms. It involves the spread of jerking movements, originally of one body part, to half the patient's body.

**Lemniscal system:** one of the two somatosensory pathways. It transmits several different types of somatosensory information, including tactile information, to the brain.

**Limbic system:** made up of the limbic lobe and areas of subcortical and cortical gray matter. Among the important structures in the limbic system are: parts of the thalamus, hypothalamus, hippocampus, and amygdala. The limbic system is especially important in the control of emotional and motivational behavior.

**Long-term memory:** a memory system in which an individual retains experiences for an extended period of time. Its capacity is very large. Long-term memory is of two varieties: generic and episodic.

**Lower motor neurons:** neurons of the motor system that originate at the brain stem or spinal cord.

**Medulla:** one of the structures in the brain stem.

**Memory trace (engram):** thought to be the consequence of subtle alterations in structural/biochemical properties of neurons as a result of learning.

**Mirror movement (overflow):** the most common type of abnormal associated movement seen in children. In mirror movement, voluntary movements on one side of the body are mirrored on the opposite side of the body. Mirror movement most often involves hand and finger movements.

**Mneumonics:** techniques developed to facilitate the process of retrieving memory trace. They employ verbal reorganization of the material and visual cues.

**Motor cortex:** region of the frontal lobe. Voluntary motor impulses originate in the motor cortex.

**Motor homunculus:** a schema of the body that is represented in the precentral gyrus of the frontal cortex. The bulk of the representation is contralateral. It is proportional to the fineness of motor control required of a body part.

**Muscle tone:** constant low level of activity, or tension, in the muscles, reflected in resistance when an individual's limb is moved passively through the range of motion.

**Myelin:** the fatty covering of neural fibers. It aids in the efficient conduction of neural impulses.

**Neonatal seizures:** type of infant and childhood seizures. They may be partial or generalized. The behavioral symptoms are usually subtle.

**Nerve cell:** see Neuron.

**Nerve deafness:** diminished sensitivity to sounds or spoken language, caused by dysfunction of the cochlear organ, the auditory nerve, or the auditory brain stem pathway. Such dysfunction typically affects a restricted frequency range, most often the high frequency range.

**Neural impulse:** an electrochemical disturbance that originates in the cell body, triggered by stimuli that are above threshold. The impulse travels along the axon of the nerve cell.

**Neuron (nerve cell):** the basic unit of the nervous system. It consists of dendrites, a cell body, and an axon.

**Nondominant:** a term that typically refers to the cerebral hemisphere (usually the right one) that is not responsible for language functions. It is also used to describe the nonpreferred hand.

**Nystagmus:** a disorder of conjugate eye movement involving involuntary rhythmical or unrhythmical oscillation of one or both eyes.

**Object agnosia:** a condition in which an individual cannot recognize a familiar stimulus (e.g., dog) despite recognition of its component parts (e.g., tail, legs, ears). He can recognize the object by smell, or touch.

**Occipital lobe:** a main subdivision of the cerebral cortex. It is responsible for the reception and processing of visual information.

**Ocular dysmetria:** a disorder of voluntary eye movement that precludes tracking a moving target or looking suddenly from one target to another.

**Ocular dyspraxia:** a disorder of voluntary eye movement that precludes voluntary turning of the eye in a given direction upon verbal command.

**Oromotor apraxia:** a disturbance in the ability to pantomime and initiate movements of the mouth and speech musculature upon verbal command. It may involve nonspeech as well speech movements.

**Paralysis:** total lack of muscle strength.

**Paraphasias:** substitutions of words that are phonetically similar (literal paraphasias) or semantically similar (verbal paraphasias) but that, in fact, have a different meaning.

**Parasympathetic system:** a subdivision of the autonomic nervous system. It facilitates vegetative functions of the body, e.g., elimination of wastes, conservation of bodily resources.

**Paresis:** partial diminution of muscle strength or weakness.

**Parietal lobe:** a principal division of the cerebral cortex. Reception and association areas for somatosensory information are located in this region. Higher association areas, responsible for the integration of intersensory information, are also in this cortical region.

**Partial (focal) seizures:** epileptic seizures localized in a part of the cerebral cortex or subcortical region. Secondary generalization occurs when focal seizure activity spreads to the entire cortex.

**Peripheral nervous (PNS) system:** made up of cranial nerves, spinal nerves, and portions of the autonomic nervous system.

**Perseveration:** a motor disturbance characterized by inappropriate repetition of a particular motor act.

**Petit mal seizures (absences):** generalized epileptic seizures lasting from one to ten seconds during which consciousness is lost.

**Plasticity:** pliability of neuronal brain tissue that allows an individual to recover functionally from central nervous system damage.

**Postictal period:** the period of time after an epileptic seizure. Characteristics of this period are a function of the type of epileptic seizure experienced. During this time some individuals become agitated. If the agitation is very severe it may be labeled postictal psychosis.

**Postural (resting) tremors:** tremors that are most prominent during rest and are initially suppressed during intented movements. As performance of a task progresses, they reemerge.

**Prefrontal cortex:** the anterior part of the frontal lobe. It is responsible for the highest level of integration of information from cortical and subcortical regions. The planning, initiation, evaluation, and modification of behavior are mediated by this cortical region.

**Premotor cortex:** the part of the frontal lobe responsible for the finely coordinated and complex motor programs that underlie skilled motor functions.

**Primary generalized seizures:** epileptic seizures that, from the start, involve the whole cortex.

**Proactive inhibition:** interference with a memory trace in which previously learned information interferes with the remembering of new information.

**Prosody:** the rhythmic or melodic intonation of speech.

**Prosopagnosia:** a visual disturbance that involves the inability to recognize familiar faces.

**Pseudoepileptic seizures:** behaviors that typically mimic tonic-clonic seizures. They are considered hysterical conversion reactions.

**Psychomotor automatisms:** behavioral abnormalities that typically occur in complex partial seizures. They are simple, habitual movements that are performed repeatedly and purposelessly. More complex automatisms rarely occur.

**Psychomotor seizures:** See Complex partial seizures.

**Pyramidal system:** one of the two motor systems that control human motor activity. It initiates, controls, and maintains voluntary motor activity via a pathway that consists of upper and lower motor neurons.

**Recent long-term memory:** information that was stored in long-term memory in the relatively recent past (minutes to months ago).

**Remote long-term memory:** information that was stored in long-term memory in the distant past.

**Reticular activating system (RAS):** an important structure in the brain stem that receives and integrates information from the senses and the cortex. The descending pathways influence selective attention; the ascending pathways mediate cortical arousal.

**Retroactive inhibition:** interference with memory functions in which new learning interferes with the remembering of old information.

**Retrograde amnesia:** a condition in which an individual is unable to retrieve experiences prior to a brain insult. It commonly follows a severe brain injury or a prolonged epileptic seizure.

**Rigidity:** a muscle tone disturbance in which excessive resistance is present throughout the range of movement, independent of the speed of manipulation.

**Sensory buffer:** the memory subsystem in which a stimulus is registered on the senses. The buffer, which is modality-specific, holds the sensation for a very short period of time after the stimulus is withdrawn.

**Sensory homunculus:** the schematic representation of the distribution of the body's somatosensory receptors located in the parietal lobe. The bulk of the representation is contralateral to the body side. The size of the representation of each body part is a function of the body part's sensitivity.

**Short-term (immediate) memory:** a memory system capable of holding a limited number of unrelated items for immediate retrieval. Items stored in short-term memory remain available for recall for approximately thirty seconds.

**Simultanagnosia:** a condition in which an individual is unable to recognize or abstract the meaning of a complex visual stimulus despite accurately perceiving its individual details.

**Soft signs:** subtle deviations in a wide range of behaviors due to brain immaturity or brain dysfunction.

**Somatic nervous system:** comprised of the sensory receptors, sensory pathways, the brain, spinal cord, motor pathways and the neuromuscular endings of the voluntary muscles in the head and body. It conveys information to the central nervous system from the body and from the central nervous system to the voluntary muscles.

**Somatosensory (sensory) cortex:** the sensory strip located in the anterior region of the parietal lobe that receives and interprets sensory information from the body. The sensory homunculus is located in this area.

**Spasticity:** a muscle tone disturbance in which the resistance of a limb throughout the range of motion increases in relation to the speed of manipulation.

**Spinal cord:** is a cylinder of gray and white matter. It has two functions: (1) it serves as a pathway and a relay station for the afferent and efferent nerves coursing to and from the brain and (2) it mediates the spinal reflexes.

**Spinal nerves:** nerves that transmit neural impulses from the sense receptors and to the muscles and glands and the body. They arise from plexi formed by the nerves that radiate from the spinal cord.

**Spinothalamic system:** one of the two somatosensory pathways. It is involved in sensations of diffuse touch, pain, and temperature.

**Status epilepticus:** the medical emergency in which complex partial and generalized epileptic seizures occur one after the other without intervening consciousness.

**Strabismus (cross-eyedness):** a disturbance of conjugate movement of the eyes in which one eye is fixated on a visual target while the other eye is directed elsewhere.

**Stuttering:** a speech disorder in which the fluency of speech is disrupted by repetitions, hesitations, and prolongations of speech sounds.

**Subcortical:** refers to brain structures that are located below the cerebral cortex.

**Sympathetic system:** a subdivision of the autonomic nervous system. It activates the organism, placing it on emergency alert.

**Synapse:** a neuronal junction within the neuronal circuit. Interneuronal communication takes place at the synapse through the release of a neurotransmitter at the presynaptic membrane. It is picked up by receptor sites on the postsynaptic membrane. Its effect on the next nerve cell may be excitatory or inhibitory.

**Temporal lobe:** a principal division of the cerebral cortex. It is responsible for the reception and processing of auditory information and, on the dominant side, mediates a number of language functions.

**Temporal lobe seizures:** see Complex partial seizures.

**Thalamus:** a subcortical structure of the nervous system. It is an important relay station for sensory information processing and part of the thalamus lies within the limbic system.

**Tics:** repetitive, stereotyped movements of single and multiple muscle groups. They commonly involve the face and neck but may also involve other body parts. They are often seen as rapid blinking, grimacing, and coughing.

**Topographical orientation defect:** the inability to describe spatial characteristics of one's environment or to orient oneself in space and on a map.

**Total auditory agnosia:** a very rare disorder that involves the inability to recognize nonspeech and speech sounds.

**Tremors:** a type of abnormal involuntary movement defined as continual rhythmic shaking of the limbs. All tremors disappear during sleep and are exacerbated by stress and anxiety. Tremors fall into two main categories: postural (resting) and intention.

**Unilateral visual neglect:** the failure to respond to stimulation in one or the other lateral visual field.

**Upper motor neurons:** the neurons in the motor system that originate at the cortical level.

**Verbal auditory agnosia (word deafness):** the inability to recognize speech sounds, despite normal hearing and preserved ability to recognize nonspeech sounds and process language that is visually presented.

**Visual agnosia:** a rare visual disorder in which an individual is unable to recognize familiar stimuli that are visually presented despite intact senstory processing, language, and general intellectual functions.

**Visual constructive disorders:** deficiencies in the ability to appreciate the spatial relations among the component parts of a visual whole and, as a consequence, deficiencies in the ability to put the parts together correctly. They may affect assembly and graphomotor tasks.

**Visual cortex:** the region of the cerebral cortex responsible for processing visual information. It is located in the occipital lobe.

**Wernicke's (sensory) aphasia:** a receptive aphasia. Its primary features are impaired comprehension of oral language and poor repetition ability.

**Wernicke's area:** located in the posterior portion of the dominant (usually left) superior temporal gyrus. It is responsible for the comprehension of oral language.

**White matter:** those regions of the nervous system composed of myelinated nerve fibers. They are called white matter because of their white color.

# Appendix 1

# DISTRIBUTORS AND PUBLISHERS OF TESTS*

American Guidance Service Inc.
Publishers' Building
Circle Pines, MN 55014

Hiskey-Nebraska Test
5640 Baldwin Ave.
Lincoln, NE 68507

Department of Psychology, Neuropsychology Clinic
University of Victoria
Victoria, British Columbia, V8W 2Y2
Canada

Pro-Ed
333 Perry Brooks Bldg.
Austin, Texas 78701

Psychological Assessment Resources Inc.
P.O. Box 996
Odessa, FL 33556

Science Research Associates Inc.
155 North Wacker Dr.
Chicago, IL 60606

The Psychological Corporation
555 Academic Ct.
San Antonio, TX 78204-0952

Western Psychological Services
12031 Wilshire Blvd.
Los Angeles, CA 90025

---

*All the tests that appear in the Appendices which follow can be obtained from one or more of the above sources.

# Appendix 2

# HISTORY*

I. Description of presenting problem
   A. Acute
      1. Onset
      2. Associated behavioral/emotional changes
      3. Possible precipitating, alleviating, and aggravating factors
   B. Recurrent
      1. Onset
      2. Associated behavioral/emotional changes
      3. Frequency, duration, changes in character of episodes
      4. Possible precipitating, alleviating, and aggravating factors

II. General description of the child
   A. Personality traits
   B. General style and level of functioning within the family
   C. Adjustment to significant life events
   D. Special interests, areas of ability, and areas of less-than-expected performance
   E. Notable behaviors and attitudes

III. Developmental history
   A. Prenatal, perinatal, and postnatal
      1. Parental reaction to pregnancy, parental relationship during pregnancy
      2. Prenatal medical care, mother's health
      3. Duration of pregnancy, type of delivery
      4. Mother's and newborn's health
   B. Childhood
      1. Place in family constellation
      2. Developmental milestones
      3. Sexual development and adjustment
      4. Significant past and current medical illnesses
      5. Previous assessment, treatment

IV. Social history
   A. Family constellation, relationships within the family
   B. Nature of past and current peer relationships, ability to sustain relationships

V. Academic history
   A. Age at time of first school experience
   B. Past and current level of academic performance and school behavior
   C. Relationships with teachers and schoolmates
   D. Previous assessments, remediation, special class placement

VI. Family history
   A. Historical and current family composition and relationships among family members
   B. Current living arrangements, financial resources, support systems
      1. Assets and weaknesses of caretakers
      2. Intrafamilial conflict

C. Significant family events, anniversaries, losses
D. Medical illnesses
E. Psychiatric disorders
F. Developmental disorders and learning problems
G. Drug and alcohol abuse
H. Child and spouse abuse

---

*The above outline is not meant to be inclusive. It is meant to serve as a guide in the development of an evaluation procedure to be modified as needed, in individual cases, by the psychologist.

# Appendix 3

# SCHOOL REPORT*

Name of Child ______________________________ Date of Birth ____________

Address ______________________________

______________________________ School ____________

Grade ____________

Teacher ____________

## ACADEMIC PERFORMANCE

### *Class Record*

Strengths (e.g., reading) ______________________________

Weaknesses (e.g., spelling) ______________________________

Approximate rank in class (e.g., lower third) ______________________________

### *Results of Standardized Testing*

*Reading:* Test ____________ Date ____________

Score (%) ____________

Class rank ____________

*Mathematics:* Test ____________ Date ____________

Score (%) ____________

Class rank ____________

*Other:* Test ____________ Date ____________

Score (%) ____________

Class rank ____________

***Academic skills***

Readiness: ______

Subskills (e.g., letter-sound associations): ______

Motor Skills (fine and gross): ______

Speech/Language: ______

***Study skills***

| *Ability to:* | *Poor* | *Fair* | *Good* | *Excellent* |
|---|---|---|---|---|
| Attend | ____ | ____ | ____ | ____ |
| Focus | ____ | ____ | ____ | ____ |
| Complete long-range assignments (e.g., book reports) | ____ | ____ | ____ | ____ |
| Complete homework | ____ | ____ | ____ | ____ |
| Work independently | ____ | ____ | ____ | ____ |
| Participate in class discussion | ____ | ____ | ____ | ____ |
| Follow class routine | ____ | ____ | ____ | ____ |
| Ask for help | ____ | ____ | ____ | ____ |
| Use help from adults/ peers | ____ | ____ | ____ | ____ |
| Organize self (e.g., desk, notebook) | ____ | ____ | ____ | ____ |
| Use reference materials (e.g., dictionary) | ____ | ____ | ____ | ____ |

Other:

______

______

______

**BEHAVIOR**

Social Skills (with adults, peers; one-to-one, group): ______________________________

Affect and emotional control: ______________________________

Conduct and behavioral control (in academic and non-academic settings): ______________

______________________________

**ADDITIONAL COMMENTS:**

Report completed by ______________________________ Date ______________________

*The above outline is meant to serve as a guide in the development of an evaluation procedure to be modified as needed, in individual cases, by the psychologist.

# Appendix 4

# CLINICAL OBSERVATION*

I. Appearance
   A. Descriptive data: age, sex, height, weight
      1. Appearance for chronological age and sex
      2. Features and behavior of note
   B. Dress
      1. Appropriateness for age, sex, and weather
      2. Condition of clothes
      3. Sloppiness or fastidiousness in dress and grooming
   C. Personal cleanliness
   D. Vegetative functions (e.g., appetite, sleep)

II. Motor activity
   A. General level and quality of activity
   B. Quality of gross motor and fine motor behavior
   C. Abnormal posturing, behavior inappropriate for age, or any other behavior of note (e.g., habit phenomena)
   D. Degree of impulse control

III. Speech and language
   A. Speech
      1. Speed and quantity
      2. Voice quality
      3. Prosody
      4. Articulation
      5. Disturbances (e.g., echolalia)
   B. Automatic language
   C. Receptive language
      1. Comprehension of questions, directions, and comments presented orally
         a. Evidence of aphasic features
   D. Expressive language
      1. Spontaneous language
         a. Amount and quality
         b. Use of language to express ideas and feelings
         c. Evidence of aphasic features
      2. Responsive language
         a. Verbal response to questions, directions, and comments
         b. Verbal expression of ideas and feelings
         c. Evidence of aphasic features

IV. Cognitive skills and general intelligence
  A. Attention span
  B. Ability to focus
  C. Memory
  D. Orientation
  E. Judgment
  F. Level of abstraction
  G. Fund of general knowledge

V. Emotional state: mood and affect
  A. General impression
    1. Range and modulation
    2. Appropriateness
    3. Congruence between mood and affect
  B. Precipitating, alleviating, or aggrevating factors around changes in emotional state

VI. Sensory experiences
  A. Extraordinary experiences (e.g., hallucinations)
  B. Disorders (e.g., agnosia)

VII. Thought characteristics
  A. Processes
    1. Speed
    2. Continuity and clarity
  B. Content
    1. Preoccupations
    2. Beliefs
    3. Experience of self, body, mood, impulses

VIII. Relatedness
  A. Eye contact
  B. Style of interaction with parents, siblings, psychologist
    1. Awareness of impact of behavior and verbalizations on others
  C. Precipitating, alleviating, or aggrevating factors around changes in relatedness

---

*The above outline is meant to serve as a guide in the development of an evaluation procedure to be modified as needed, in individual cases, by the psychologist.

The following Appendices are meant to serve as a guide in the development of an evaluation procedure to be modified as needed, in individual cases, by the psychologist.

Certain measures are not part of the routine comprehensive psychological evaluation either because: they do not exist; they are not routinely used; or because the assessment of the skill is not within the domain of the psychologist.

# Appendix 5

# REPRESENTATIVE QUANTITATIVE AND QUALITATIVE MEASURES OF LANGUAGE COMPETENCE, LANGUAGE SUBSKILLS, AND SPEECH

**Language**

**Competence**

- Quantitative
  - McCarthy: Verbal subtests
  - WISC-R: Verbal subtests
- Qualitative
  - Developmental history
  - School report
  - Features of test performance
  - Automatic, receptive, and expressive language

**Subskills: Specific Features and Neuropsychological Functions**

- Quantitative
  - ITPA: Auditory Sequential Memory
  - NCCEA
  - Wepman
- Qualitative
  - Developmental history
  - School report
  - Features of test performance
  - Automatic, receptive, and expressive language

**Speech**

- Quantitative
  - NCCEA: Articulation
  - Pantomime of buccofacial movements on verbal command
- Qualitative
  - Developmental history
  - School report
  - Features of test performance
  - Automatic and expressive language

---

**Key**—ITPA: Illinois Test of Psycholinguistic Abilities
McCarthy: McCarthy Scale of Children's Abilities
NCCEA: Neurosensory Center Comprehensive Examination for Aphasia
Wepman: Wepman Auditory Word Discrimination Test
WISC-R: Wechsler Intelligence Scale for Children–Revised

# Appendix 6

# REPRESENTATIVE QUANTITATIVE AND QUALITATIVE MEASURES OF MEMORY

**Short-Term Memory**

- Auditory
  - Quantitative
    - ITPA: Auditory Sequential Memory
    - NCCEA: Digit Forward, Digit Backward, Sentence Repetition
    - WISC-R: Digit Span
  - Qualitative
    - Intertest performance variability
    - Receptive and expressive language
- Visual
  - Quantitative
    - Benton
    - H-N: Memory for Color, Visual Attention Span
    - ITPA: Visual Sequential Memory
  - Qualitative
    - Features of test performance
    - Memory "tricks"

**Long-Term Memory**

- Quantitative*
- Qualitative
  - Academic history
  - School report
  - Response to series of simple commands
  - Fund of general information

---

**Key**—Benton: Benton Visual Retention Test–Revised
H-N: Hiskey Nebraska Test of Learning Aptitude
ITPA: Illinois Test of Psycholinguistic Abilities
NCCEA: Neurosensory Center Comprehensive Examination for Aphasia
WISC–R: Wechsler Intelligence Scale for Children–Revised

* Not part of routine comprehensive psychological evaluation.

# Appendix 7

# REPRESENTATIVE QUANTITATIVE AND QUALITATIVE MEASURES OF VISUAL DISORDERS

**Visual Acuity Disorder**

- Quantitative*
- Qualitative
  - Distance visual material is held from face

**Ocular Motility Disorder**

- Quantitative
  - Tracking task
- Qualitative
  - Features of test performance
  - Response pattern on visual tasks
  - Position and activity of the eyes at rest and during visual tasks

**Visual Field Defect**

- Quantitative*
- Qualitative
  - Position of the head during visual tasks

**Visual Information Processing Disorder**

- Perceptual
  - Quantitative
    - H-N: Completion of Drawings
    - ITPA: Visual Closure
    - Ravens
  - Qualitative
    - Features of test performance
- Visual spatial
  - Quantitative*
  - Qualitative
    - Response to the visual field
- Visual Constructive
  - Quantitative
    - Benton
    - McCarthy: Block Building, Puzzle Solving
    - V-MI
    - WISC-R: Block Design, Object Assembly, Coding

Qualitative
- Academic history
- School report
- Features of test performance
- Intertest performance variability
- Graphomotor and assembly task performance

---

**Key**—Benton: Benton Visual Retention Test–Revised
H-N: Hiskey Nebraska Test of Learning Aptitude
ITPA: Illinois Test of Psycholinguistic Abilities
McCarthy: McCarthy Scales of Children's Abilities
Ravens: Ravens Coloured and Standard Progressive Matrices
V-MI: Developmental Test of Visual-Motor Integration
WISC-R: Wechsler Intelligence Scale for Children–Revised

*Not part of routine comprehensive psychological evaluation.

# Appendix 8

# REPRESENTATIVE QUANTITATIVE AND QUALITATIVE MEASURES OF AUDITORY DISORDERS

**Deafness**

**Conductive (Transmission)**

- Quantitative*
- Qualitative
  - Receptive and expressive language
  - Speech

**Nerve**

- Quantitative*
- Qualitative
  - As in conductive (transmission) deafness

**Auditory Discrimination Disorder**

- Quantitative
  - G-F-W
  - Wepman
- Qualitative
  - Discrimination of similar nonspeech sounds
  - Discrimination of similar speech sounds
  - Speech

**Auditory Agnosia**

- Quantitative*
- Qualitative
  - Recognition of familiar nonspeech sounds
  - Recognition of familiar speech sounds

---

**Key**—G-F-W: Goldman-Fristoe-Woodcock Test of Auditory Discrimination
Wepman: Wepman Auditory Discrimination Test

*Not part of routine comprehensive psychological evaluation

# Appendix 9

# REPRESENTATIVE QUANTITATIVE AND QUALITATIVE MEASURES OF TOUCH AND BODY SCHEMA DISORDERS

**Touch**

**Tactile Localization Disorder**

Quantitative*
Qualitative*

**Two-Point Discrimination Disorder**

Quantitative*
Qualitative*

**Double Simultaneous Discrimination Disorder**

Quantitative*
Qualitative*

**Agraphesthesia**

Quantitative
- Recognition of familiar shapes, numbers, or letters "written" on the hand

Qualitative
- Features of test performance

**Haptic Imperception**

Quantitative
- NCCEA: Tactile Visual Matching

Qualitative
- Features of test performance

**Astereognosis**

Quantitative
- NCCEA: Tactile Naming

Qualitative
- Features of test performance

**Body Schema**

**Finger Agnosia**

Quantitative
- Tactile recognition of fingers

Qualitative
- Features of test performance
- Finger counting

### Right-Left Disorientation

Quantitative
  McCarthy: Right-left Orientation
Qualitative
  Receptive and expressive language

### Gerstmann Syndrome

Quantitative
  As in finger agnosia, right-left disorientation, writing disorder, and arithmetic disorder
Qualitative
  As in finger agnosia, right-left disorientation, writing disorder, and arithmetic disorder

### Neglect

Quantitative*
Qualitative
  Developmental history
  Activities of daily living

---

**Key**—McCarthy: McCarthy Scales of Children's Abilities
NCCEA: Neurosensory Center Comprehensive Examination for Aphasia

*Not part of routine comprehensive psychological evaluation

# Appendix 10

# REPRESENTATIVE QUANTITATIVE AND QUALITATIVE MEASURES OF MOTOR DISORDERS

**Tone Disorder**

- Quantitative*
- Qualitative
  - Fine motor tasks
  - Gross motor tasks

**Strength Disorder**

- Quantitative*
- Qualitative
  - Fine motor tests
  - Gross motor tests

**Coordination Disorder**

- Fine Motor
  - Quantitative
    - Finger manipulation tests
    - Purdue
    - V-MI
  - Qualitative
    - Developmental history
    - School report
    - Features of test performance
    - Fine motor tasks
- Gross Motor
  - Quantitative
    - McCarthy: Leg Coordination
  - Qualitative
    - Developmental history
    - School report
    - Features of test performance
    - Gross motor tasks

**Abnormal Involuntary Movements**

- Quantitative*
- Qualitative
  - Presence of tics or tremors

**Abnormal Associated Movements**

- Quantitative*
- Qualitative
  - Overflow to mouth or to opposing hand

**Learned Skilled Motor Act Disorder**

- Ideomotor
  - Quantitative
    - Pantomime of simple acts on verbal command
  - Qualitative
    - Features of test performance
- Ideational
  - Quantitative
    - Pantomime of complex acts on verbal command
  - Qualitative
    - Features of test performance

**Perseveration**

- Quantitative*
- Qualitative
  - Perseverative test responses, verbal or nonverbal
  - Perseverative spontaneous behavior, verbal or nonverbal

---

**Key**—McCarthy: McCarthy Scales of Children's Abilities
Purdue: Purdue Pegboard Test
V-MI: Developmental Test of Visual-Motor Integration

*Not part of routine comprehensive psychological evaluation

# Appendix 11

# REPRESENTATIVE QUANTITATIVE AND QUALITATIVE MEASURES OF READING COMPETENCE

**Decoding**

Single Word

- Quantitative
  - R-C
  - WRAT-R
  - WRMT: Word Attack
- Qualitative
  - School report
  - Features of test performance
  - Decoding tests

Sequential Reading

- Quantitative
  - Gilmore
  - Gray-R
- Qualitative
  - Academic history
  - School report
  - Features of test performance
  - Decoding tasks

**Comprehension**

Single Word

- Quantitative
  - WRMT: Word Comprehension
- Qualitative
  - Features of test performance
  - Comprehension tests

Sequential Reading

- Quantitative
  - Gray-R
  - WRMT: Passage Comprehension
- Qualitative
  - Academic history
  - School report
  - Features of test performance

**Key**—Gilmore: Gilmore Oral Reading Test
Gray-R: Gray Oral Reading Test-Revised
R-C: Roswell-Chall Diagnostic Reading Test
WRAT-R: Wide Range Achievement Test–Revised
WRMT: Woodcock Reading Mastery Test

# Appendix 12

# REPRESENTATIVE QUANTITATIVE AND QUALITATIVE MEASURES OF READING SUBSKILLS

**Sensory Acuity**

- Visual
  - Quantitative*
  - Qualitative
    - Distance visual material is held from face
- Auditory
  - Quantitative*
  - Qualitative
    - Receptive and expressive language
    - Speech
- Somatosensory
  - Quantitative*
  - Qualitative
    - Fine motor tasks

**Perceptual Discrimination**

- Visual
  - Quantitative
    - Ravens
  - Qualitative
    - Features of test performance
    - Reports of visual confusion
- Auditory
  - Quantitative
    - G-F-W
    - Seashore
    - Wepman
  - Qualitative
    - Features of test performance
    - Receptive and expressive language
    - Speech
- Somatosensory
  - Quantitative*
  - Qualitative
    - Fine motor tasks

**Visual Memory**

- Quantitative
  - Benton
  - ITPA: Visual Sequential Memory
  - McCarthy: Pictorial Memory
- Qualitative
  - Features of test performance
  - Intertest performance variability

**Auditory Memory**

- Quantitative
  - ITPA: Auditory Sequential Memory
  - McCarthy: Verbal Memory 1, Verbal Memory 2
  - NCCEA: Digits Forward, Digits Backward, Sentence Repetition
- Qualitative
  - Features of test performance
  - Intertest performance variability
  - Recall of names of significant people
  - Fund of general knowledge

**Grapheme-Phoneme Associations**

- Quantitative
  - R-C
- Qualitative
  - Academic history
  - School report
  - Features of test performance
  - Decoding tasks

**Word-Label Associations**

- Quantitative
  - Gilmore
  - R-C
  - WRAT-R
- Qualitative
  - Academic history
  - School report
  - Features of test performance
  - Decoding tasks

**Segmenting Skills**

- Quantitative*
- Qualitative
  - Decoding tasks

**Conditional Learning**

- Quantitative*
- Qualitative
  - Decoding tasks

**Modality Shift**

- Quantitative*
- Qualitative
  - Decoding tasks

**Sound Blending**

- Quantitative
  - ITPA: Sound Blending
- Qualitative
  - School report
  - Features of test performance

**Ocular Motility**

- Quantitative
  - Tracking task
- Qualitative
  - Features of test performance
  - Position and activity of the eyes during visual tasks

**Left-to-Right Work Pattern**

- Quantitative*
- Qualitative
  - Work patterns on visual tasks

**Strategy Shift**

- Quantitative*
- Qualitative
  - Decoding tasks

**Spatial Orientation**

- Quantitative*
- Qualitative
  - Decoding tasks

**Somatosensory Memory**

- Quantitative*
- Qualitative
  - Fine motor tasks

**Oral Praxis**

- Quantitative
  - NCCEA: Articulation
  - Pantomime of buccofacial movements on verbal command
- Qualitative
  - Features of test performance
  - Automatic and expressive language

**Grammatical Markings**

- Quantitative*
- Qualitative
  - Sequential reading tasks

**Language Skills**

- Quantitative
  - NCCEA
  - WISC-R: Verbal subtests
- Qualitative
  - Developmental history
  - School report
  - Receptive and expressive language

**General Intelligence**

- Quantitative
  - WISC-R: Verbal subtests
- Qualitative
  - Fund of general knowledge

---

**Key**—Benton: Benton Visual Retention Test–Revised
Gilmore: Gilmore Oral Reading Test
G-F-W: Goldman-Fristoe-Woodcock Test of Auditory Discrimination
Gray-R: Gray Oral Reading Test-Revised
ITPA: Illinois Test of Psycholinguistic Abilities
McCarthy: McCarthy Scales of Children's Abilities
NCCEA: Neurosensory Center Comprehensive Examination for Aphasia
Ravens: Ravens Coloured and Standard Progressive Matrices
R-C: Roswell-Chall Diagnostic Reading Test
Seashore: Seashore Rhythm Test
WISC-R: Wechsler Intelligence Scale for Children–Revised
WRAT-R: Wide Range Achievement Test–Revised
WRMT: Woodcock Reading Mastery Test

*Not part of routine comprehensive psychological evaluation

# Appendix 13

# REPRESENTATIVE QUANTITATIVE AND QUALITATIVE MEASURES OF WRITING COMPETENCE

**Single Word**

- Quantitative
  - TOWL: Spelling
  - WRAT-R: Spelling
- Qualitative
  - Academic history
  - School report
  - Features of test performance
  - Automatic spelling

**Sentences**

- Quantitative
  - TOWL
- Qualitative
  - School report
  - Features of test performance
  - Writing tasks

---

**Key**—TOWL: Test of Written Language
WRAT-R: Wide Range Achievement Test–Revised

# Appendix 14

# REPRESENTATIVE QUANTITATIVE AND QUALITATIVE MEASURES OF WRITING SUBSKILLS

**Sensory Acuity**

- Visual
  - Quantitative*
  - Qualitative
    - Distance visual material is held from face
- Auditory
  - Quantitative*
  - Qualitative
    - Receptive and expressive language
    - Speech
- Somatosensory
  - Quantitative*
  - Qualitative
    - Fine motor tasks

**Perceptual Discrimination**

- Visual
  - Quantitative
    - Ravens
  - Qualitative
    - Features of test performance
    - Reports of visual confusion
- Auditory
  - Quantitative
    - G-F-W
    - Seashore
    - Wepman
  - Qualitative
    - Features of test performance
    - Receptive and expressive language
    - Speech
- Somatosensory
  - Quantitative
    - Recognition of familiar shapes, numbers, or letter "written" on the hand
    - Tactile recognition of fingers
  - Qualitative
    - Features of test performance

**Segmenting Skills**

Quantitative*
Qualitative
Writing tasks

**Auditory Memory**

Quantitative
ITPA: Auditory Sequential Memory
McCarthy: Verbal Memory 1, Verbal Memory 2
NCCEA: Digits Forward, Digits Backward, Sentence Repetition
Qualitative
Intertest performance variability
Response to series of simple commands
Recall of names of significant people

**Visual Memory**

Quantitative
Benton
H-N: Memory for Color, Attention Span
ITPA: Visual Sequential Memory
Qualitative
Features of test performance
Intertest performance variability

**Phoneme-Grapheme Associations**

Quantitative*
Qualitative
Writing tasks
Direct testing of sound-letter associations

**Conditional Learning**

Quantitative*
Qualitative
Writing tasks

**Oral Word-Visual Image Associations**

Quantitative
TOWL: Spelling
WRAT-R: Spelling
Qualitative
Academic history
School report
Writing tasks
Automatic spelling

**Modality Shift**

Quantitative*
Qualitative
Writing tasks

**Strategy Shift**

Quantitative*
Qualitative
Writing tasks

**Left-to-Right Work Pattern**

Quantitative*
Qualitative
Writing tasks
Work patterns on visual tasks

**Somatosensory Memory**

Quantitative*
Qualitative
Writing tasks
Fine motor tasks

**Fine Motor Coordination**

Quantitative
Purdue
Finger manipulation tests
Qualitative
Features of test performance
Fine motor tasks

**Graphomotor Skills**

Quantitative
Bender
Benton
TOWL: Handwriting
V-MI
Qualitative
Features of test performance
Graphomotor tasks

**Spatial Orientation**

Quantitative*
Qualitative
Writing tasks

**Spatial Organization**

Quantitative
Bender
Benton
V-MI

Qualitative
  Features of test performance
  Writing tasks

**Grammatical Markings**

Quantitative
  TOWL: Style
Qualitative
  Features of test performance
  Writing tasks

**Oral Praxis**

Quantitative
  NCCEA: Articulation
  Pantomime of buccofacial movements on verbal command
Qualitative
  Features of test performance
  Automatic and expressive language

**Language Skills**

Quantitative
  NCCEA
  TOWL: Vocabulary, Thematic Maturity
  WISC-R: Verbal subtests
Qualitative
  Receptive and expressive language

**General Intelligence**

Quantitative
  WISC-R: Verbal subtests
Qualitative
  Fund of general knowledge

---

**Key**—Bender: Bender Visual Motor Gestalt Test
Benton: Benton Visual Retention Test–Revised
G-F-W: Goldman-Fristoe-Woodcock Auditory Discrimination Test
H-N: Hiskey Nebraska Test of Learning Aptitude
ITPA: Illinois Test of Psycholinguistic Abilities
McCarthy: McCarthy Scales of Children's Abilities
NCCEA: Neurosensory Center Comprehensive Examination for Aphasia
Purdue: Purdue Pegboard
Ravens: Ravens Coloured and Standard Progressive Matrices
Seashore: Seashore Rhythm Test
TOWL: Test of Written Language
V-MI: Beery-Bukentica Visual-Motor Integration Test
WISC-R: Wechsler Intelligence Scale for Children–Revised
WRAT-R: Wide Range Achievement Test–Revised

*Not part of routine comprehensive psychological evaluation

# Appendix 15

# REPRESENTATIVE QUANTITATIVE AND QUALITATIVE MEASURES OF ARITHMETIC COMPETENCE

**Number Counting and Comprehension**

- Quantitative
  - McCarthy: Arithmetic
  - WISC-R: Arithmetic
  - WRAT-R: Arithmetic
- Qualitative
  - Rote counting
  - Receptive and expressive language
  - Spontaneous behavior

**Arithmetic Calculation**

- Quantitative
  - McCarthy: Arithmetic
  - WISC-R: Arithmetic
  - WRAT-R: Arithmetic
- Qualitative
  - Academic history
  - School report
  - Features of test performance
  - Intertest performance variability

**Numerical Problem Solving**

- Quantitative
  - WISC-R: Arithmetic
  - WRAT-R: Arithmetic
- Qualitative
  - School report
  - Features of test performance

---

**Key**—McCarthy: McCarthy Scales of Children's Abilities
WISC-R: Wechsler Intelligence Scale for Children–Revised
WRAT–R: Wide Range Achievement Test–Revised

# Appendix 16

# REPRESENTATIVE QUANTITATIVE AND QUALITATIVE MEASURES OF ARITHMETIC SUBSKILLS

**Sensory Acuity**

- Visual
  - Quantitative*
  - Qualitative
    - Distance visual material is held from face
- Auditory
  - Quantitative*
  - Qualitative
    - Receptive and expressive language
    - Speech
- Somatosensory
  - Quantitative*
  - Qualitative
    - Fine motor tasks

**Perceptual Discrimination**

- Visual
  - Quantitative
    - Ravens
  - Qualitative
    - Features of test performance
    - Reports of visual confusion
- Auditory
  - Quantitative
    - G-F-W
    - Seashore
    - Wepman
  - Qualitative
    - Features of test performance
    - Receptive and expressive language
    - Speech
- Somatosensory
  - Quantitative
    - Recognition of familiar shapes, numbers, or letters "written" on the hand
    - Tactile recognition of fingers
  - Qualitative
    - Features of test performance

**Visual Memory**

- Quantitative
  - Benton
  - H-N: Memory for Color, Visual Attention Span
  - ITPA: Visual Sequential Memory
  - McCarthy: Pictorial Memory
- Qualitative
  - Features of test performance
  - Memory "tricks"
  - Intertest performance variability

**Auditory Memory**

- Quantitative
  - ITPA: Auditory Sequential Memory
  - McCarthy: Verbal Memory 1, Verbal Memory 2
  - NCCEA: Digits Forward, Digits Backward, Sentence Repetition
- Qualitative
  - Features of test performance
  - Intertest performance variability
  - Response to series of simple commands

**Somatosensory Memory**

- Quantitative*
- Qualitative
  - Writing tasks
  - Fine motor tasks

**Modality Shift**

- Quantitative*
- Qualitative
  - Enumeration tasks

**Fine Motor Coordination**

- Quantitative
  - Purdue
  - Finger manipulation tests
- Qualitative
  - School report
  - Features of test performance
  - Fine motor tasks

**One-to-One Correspondence**

- Quantitative
  - WISC-R: Arithmetic
  - WRAT-R: Arithmetic
- Qualitative
  - Features of test performance
  - Counting tasks

**Work pattern**

- Quantitative*
- Qualitative
    - Calculation tasks

**Comprehension of Number Value**

- Quantitative
    - WISC-R: Arithmetic
    - WRAT-R: Arithmetic
- Qualitative
    - Features of test performance
    - Counting tasks

**Conceptual Development**

- Quantitative
    - NCCEA: Token test
- Qualitative
    - Receptive and expressive language
    - Spontaneous behavior

**Verbal-Visual (Number) Associations**

- Quantitative*
- Qualitative
    - Number dictation tasks

**Verbal-Visual (Sign) Associations**

- Quantitative*
- Qualitative
    - Dictated calculation tasks

**Verbal/Visual-Operation Associations**

- Quantitative
    - WRAT-R: Arithmetic
- Qualitative
    - School report
    - Features of test performance

**Operation Procedures**

- Quantitative
    - WISC-R: Arithmetic
    - WRAT-R: Arithmetic
- Qualitative
    - School report
    - Features of test performance

**Number Facts**

- Qualitative*

Quantitative
- School report
- Calculation tasks

**Graphomotor Skills**

Quantitative
- Bender
- Benton
- V-MI

Qualitative
- School report
- Features of test performance
- Graphomotor tasks

**Spatial Orientation**

Quantitative*

Qualitative
- Written calculations tasks

**Spatial Organization**

Quantitative
- Bender
- Benton
- V-MI

Qualitative
- Feature of test performance
- Written calculation tasks

**Oral Praxis**

Quantitative
- NCCEA: Articulation
- Pantomime of buccofacial movements on verbal command

Qualitative
- Features of test performance
- Automatic and expressive language

**Reading Competence**

Quantitative
- Gilmore
- WRMT: Passage Comprehension

Qualitative
- School report
- Features of test performance

**Language Skills**

Quantitative
- NCCEA
- WISC-R: Verbal subtests

Qualitative

Receptive and expressive language

**General Intelligence**

Quantitative

WISC-R: Verbal subtests

Qualitative

Fund of general knowledge

---

**Key**—Bender: Bender Visual Motor Gestalt Test
Benton: Benton Visual Retention Test– Revised
G-F-W: Goldman-Fristoe-Woodcock Auditory Discrimination Test
H-N: Hiskey Nebraska Test of Learning Aptitude
ITPA: Illinois Test of Psycholinguistic Abilities
McCarthy: McCarthy Scales of Children's Abilities
NCCEA: Neurosensory Center Comprehensive Examination for Aphasia
Purdue: Purdue Pegboard
Ravens: Ravens Coloured and Standard Progressive Matrices
Seashore: Seashore Rhythm Test
V-MI: Beery-Bukentica Visual-Motor Integration Test
Wepman: Wepman Auditory Discrimination Test
WISC-R: Wechsler Intelligence Test for Children-Revised
WRAT-R: Wide Range Achievement Test-Revised
WRMT: Woodcock Reading Mastery Test

*Not part of routine comprehensive psychological evaluation

# SELECTED READINGS*


### General Reference

Cummings, J. L. (1985). Clinical Neuropsychiatry. New York: Grune & Stratton.

Filskow, S. B., & Boll, T. (Eds.) (1981). Handbook of Chemical Neuropsychology. New York: John Wiley and Sons.

Heilman, K. M., & Valenstein, E. (Eds.) (1985). Clinical Neuropsychology, ed. 2. New York: Oxford University Press.

Hynd, G. W., & Obrzut, J. E. (Eds.) (1981). Neuropsychological Assessment and the School-Age Child: Issues and procedures. New York: Grune & Stratton.

Luria, A. R. (1980). Higher Cortical Functions in Man. New York: Basic Books.

Luria, A. R. (1973). The Working Brain. New York: Basic Books.

Rapin, I. (1982). Children with Brain Dysfunction: Neurology, Cognition, Language, and Behavior. New York: Raven Press.

Rourke, B. P., Bakker, D. J., Fisk, J. L., & Strong, J. D. (1983). Child Neuropsychology: An Introduction to Theory, Research, and Clinical Practice. New York: Guilford Press.

Rutter, M. (Ed.) (1983) Developmental Neuropsychiatry. New York: Guilford Press.

### Human Nervous System and Topics for Special Consideration

Aram, D. M., Ekelman, B. L., Rose, D. F., & Whitcher, H. A. (1985). Verbal and cognitive sequelae following unilateral lesions acquired in early childhood. Journal of Clinical and Experimental Neuropsychology, 7, 55-78.

Bogen, J. E. (1969). The other side of the brain II: An appositional mind. Bulletin of the Los Angeles Neurological Society, 34, 135-162.

Bogen, J. E,. & Bogen, G. M. (1969). The other side of the brain III: The corpus callosum and creativity. Bulletin of the Los Angeles Neurological Society, 34, 191-220.

Child Development (1987). Special Section: Developmental Psychology and the Neurosciences: Building a Bridge. Child Development, 58, 533-724.

Galaburda, A. M., LeMay, M., Kemper, T. L., & Geschwind, N. (1978). Right-left asymmetries in the human brain. Science, 199, 852-856.

Geschwind, N. (1965). Disconnection syndromes in animals and man. Brain, 88, 237-294, 585-644.

Hardyck, C., & Petrinovich, L. F. (1977). Left-handedness. Psychological Bulletin, F4, 385-400.

Noback, C. R., & Demarest, R. J. (1986). The Nervous System: Introduction and Review, ed. 3. New York: McGraw-Hill.

Penfield, W., & Rasmussen, T. (1955). The Cerebral Cortex of Man. New York: Macmillan.

Scientific American (1979). Special Issue on the Brain. Scientific American, 241, 45-232.

Ullman, d. G. (1977). Children's lateral preference patterns: Frequency and relationships with achievement and intelligence. Journal of School Psychiatry, 15, 36-43.

### Language Disorders

Aram, D. M., & Nation, J. E. (1975). Patterns of language behavior in children with developmental language disorder. Journal of Speech and Hearing Research, 18, 229-241.

Benton, A. L. (1964). Developmental aphasia and brain damage. Cortex, 1, 40-52.

Eisenson, J. (1972). Aphasia in Children. New York: Harper & Row.

Geschwind, N. (1974). Disorders of higher critical function in children. In N. Geshwind (Ed.), Selected Papers on Language and the Brain. Boston: Reidel.
Geschwind, N. (1972). Language and the brain. Scientific American, 226, 76-83.
Rapin, I., & Wilson, B. C. (1978). Children with developmental language disability: Neurologic aspects and assessment. In M. A. Wyke (Ed.), Developmental Dyslexia. London: Academic Press.
Schery, T. K. (1985). Correlates of language development in language-disordered children. Journal of Speech and Hearing Disorders, 50, 73-83.
Wiegel-Crump, C. A. & Dennis, M. (1986). Development of word-finding. Brain and Language, 27, 1-23.
Wilson, B. C., & Wilson, J. J. (1978). Language disordered children: A neuropsychologic view. In B. A. Fiengold & C. L. Bank (Eds.), Developmental Disabilities of Early Childhood. Springfield, IL: Charles C. Thomas.

### *Episodic Disorders: Seizures and Headaches*

Brown, J. K. (1977). Migraine and migraine equivalents in children. Developmental Medicine and Child Neurology, 19, 683-692.
Delgado-Escuela, A. V., Mattson, R. H., King, L., Goldensohn, E. S., Spiegel, H., Madson, J., Crandall, P., Dreifuss, F., and Porter, R. J. (1981). The nature of aggression during epileptic seizures. New England Journal of Medicine, 305, 711-716.
Friedman, A. P., & Harms, E. (1967). Headaches in Children. Springfield, IL: Charles C. Thomas.
Goodyer, I. M. (1985). Epileptic and pseudo-epileptic seizures in childhood and adolescence. Journal of the American Academy of Child Psychiatry, 24, 3-9.
Oktahara, J. (1984). Seizure disorders in infancy and childhood. Brain and Development, 6, 509-519.
Penfield, W., and Jasper, H. (1954). Epilepsy and the Functional Anatomy of the Human Brain. Boston: Little, Brown.
Williams, D. (1956). The structure of emotions reflected in epileptic experiences. Brain, 79, 29-67.

### *Memory Disorders*

Barbizet, J. (1970). Human Memory and Its Pathology. San Francisco: W. H. Freeman.
Gunnison, J. (1984). The role of short-term memory in the comprehension of written text. Journal of Educational Neuropsychology, 3, 19-26.
Hácaen, H., Tzortzis, C., & Rondot, P. (1980). Loss of topographic memory with learning deficits. Cortex, 16, 525-542.
Miller, G. A. (1956). The magical number seven, plus or minus two: Some limits in our capacity for processing information. Psychological Review, 63, 81-97.
Senf, G. M., and Freundl, P. C. (1971). Memory and attention factors in specific learning disabilities. Journal of Learning Disabilities, 4, 94-106.

### *Sensory and Motor Disorders*

Benton, A. L., Leven, H. S., & Van Allen, M. W. (1974). Geographic orientation in patients with unilateral cerebral disease. Neuropsychologia, 12, 183-191.
Benton, A. L., & Van Allen, M. W. (1972). Prosopagnosia and facial discrimination. Journal of Neurological Sciences, 15, 167-172.
Denkla, M. B. (1974). Development of coordination in normal children. Developmental Medicine and Child Neurology, 16, 729-741.
Gerstmann, J. (1940). Syndrome of finger agnosia, disorientation for right and left, agraphia, and acalculia. Archives of Neurology and Psychiatry, 44, 398-408.
Geschwind, N. (1975) The apraxias: Neural mechanisms of disorders of learned movement. American Scientist, 63, 188-195.
Kinsbourne, M., & Warrington, E. K. (1963). The developmental Gerstmann syndrome. Archives of Neurology, 8, 490-501.

### *Disorders of Reading, Writing, and Arithmetic*

Benson, D. F. (1984). Alexia and the neural basis of reading. Annals of Dyslexia, 34, 3-14.
Boder, E. (1973). Developmental dyslexia: A diagnostic approach based on three atypical reading-spelling patterns. Developmental Medicine and Child Neurology, 15, 663-687.
Bogen, J. E. (1969). The other side of the brain I: Dysgraphia and dyscopia following cerebral commissurotomy. Bulletin of the Los Angeles Neurological Society, 34, 73-105.
Denckla, M. B. (1977). The neurological basis of reading disability. In F. G. Rozwell & G. Natchez (Eds.), Reading Disability: A Human Approach to Learning. New York: Basic Books.
Ellis, A. W. (1985). The cognitive neuropsychology of developmental (and acquired) dyslexia: A critical survey. Cognitive Neuropsychology, 2, 169-205.
Grewel, F. (1952). Acalculia. Brain, 75, 397-407.
Henderson, V. W. (1986). Anatomy of posterior pathways in reading: A reassessment. Brain and Language, 29, 119-133.
Hynd, G. W., & Cohen, M. (1983). Dyslexia: Neuropsychological Theory, Research, and Clinical Differentiation. New York: Grune & Stratton.
Mattis, S. (1978). Dyslexia syndromes: A working hypothesis that works. In A. L. Benton & D. Pearl (Eds.), Dyslexia: An Appraisal of Current Knowledge. New York: Oxford University Press.
Nelson, H. E., & Warrington, E. K. (1976). Developmental spelling retardation. In R. M. Knights & D. J. Bakkher (Eds.), The Neuropsychology of Learning Disorders. Baltimore: University Park Press.
Pirozzolo, F. J., & Wiltrock, M. C. (Eds.) (1981). Neuropsychological and Cognitive Processes in Reading. New York: Academic Press.
Roeltgen, D. P., Cordell, C., & Sevush, S. (October 31, 1983). A battery of linguistic analysis for writing and reading. International Neuropsychological Society Bulletin.
Spellacy, F. & Peter, B. (1978). Dyscalculia and elements of the developmental Gerstmann syndrome in school children. Cortex, 14, 197-206.

### *Emotional and Behavorial Disorders*

Benton, A. L. (1968). Differential effects of frontal lobe disease. Neuropsychologia, 6, 53-60.
Hebb, D. O., & Penfield, W. (1940). Human behavior after extensive bilateral removal from the frontal lobes. Archives of Neurology and Psychiatry, 44, 421-438.
Heilman, K. M., & Satz, P. (Eds.) (1983). Neuropsychology of Human Emotion. New York: Guilford Press.
Heilman, K. M., Bowers, D., Speedie, L. S., & Coslett, H. B. (1984). Comprehension of affective and nonaffective prosody. Neurology, 34, 917-921.
Kinsbourne, M. (1977). The mechanism of hyperactivity. In M. E. Blaw, I. Rapin, & M. Kinsbourne (Eds.), Topics in Child Neurology. New York: Spectrum.
Leventhal, H. & Tomarken, A. J. (1986). Emotion: Today's problems. Annual Review of Psychology, 37, 565-610.
Ross, D. M., & Ross, S. A. (1976). Hyperactivity: Research, Theory, and Action. New York: John Wiley & Sons.
Rutter, M., & Scholper, E. (Eds.) (1978). Autism: A Reappraisal of Concepts and Treatment. New York: Plenum Press.
Schaffer, D., Schonfeld, I., O'Connor, P. A., Stokman, C., Trautman, P., Shaffer, S., & Ng, S. (1985). Neurological soft signs: Their relationship to psychiatric disorder and intelligence in childhood and adolescence. Archives of General Psychiatry, 442, 342-351.
Silberman, E. K., & Weingartner, H. (1986). Hemispheric lateralization of functions related to emotion. Brain and Cognition, 5, 322-353.

---

*The selected reading list is not inclusive. Its purpose is to provide both further information about the topics discussed in the book and to expose the reader to some classic work in the area, as well as some current writings. In addition, it offers an introduction to the breadth of investigative interests in the area.

# INDEX


Absence seizures, 56
Abstraction abilities disturbance, 143
Acalculia, 132
  with alexia or agraphia, 133
  primary, 133
  secondary, 133
Acetylcholine, 8
  emotion and, 142
Adaptive functioning, 32
Adjustment disorders, 149
Affective disorders, 14
Afferent nerve fibers, 8
  pathways of, 24–25
Age, and brain dysfunction, 28
Agnosia
  auditory, 86, 87
    causes of, 89
  color, 81
  finger, 94–95
  verbal auditory, 45
  visual, 80–81, 116
Agraphesthesia, 12, 93
Agraphia, 36, 113, 116
  with aphasia, 124–125
  apraxic, 126
  for numbers, 133
  pure, 124
  spatial, 125–126
Alexia, 36, 114–115
  with agraphia, *113*, 116
  without agraphia, *113*, 115
Ambidexterity, 32
Amnesia, 71–72
  anterograde, 73
  retrograde, 72
Angular gyrus, 9
  damage of, 112–113
Anomia, 115
Anomic aphasias, 39
Anterograde amnesia, 73
Anticonvulsants, side effects of, 60*t*
Anxiety, 150
  disorders of, 148
Aphasias. *See also specific types of.*
  with agraphia, 124–125
  classification of, 36–37
  conduction, 125
  expressive, 125
  principal features of, 38*t*
  reading disorder in, 112
  receptive, 125
  types of, 38–39
Apraxias, 49, 105–106, 126
  oromotor, 117
Apraxic agraphia, 126
Apraxic speech disorders, 49
Arithmetic competence. *See also* Calculation ability.
  assessment of, 136
  representative quantitative and qualitative measure of, 196
  neuroanatomical basis of, 132
Arithmetic disorders
  clinical syndromes of, 132–135
  diagnosis of, 135–137
  errors made in, 134–135
  historical background of, 131–132
Arithmetic subskills, 135–136
  assessment of, 136–137
  representative quantitative and qualitative measure of, 197–201
Arousal, 140–141, 150
  emotional/behavioral disorders and, 143
Articulation disorders, 48
Articulation errors, 49
Associated movements, abnormal, 105
  causes of, 107
Association cortex, 12–13, 14
  arithmetic competence and, 132
  emotion and, 140
  writing skills and, 123
Association fibers, 8–9
Astereognosis, 93
Attention-deficit hyperactivity disorders, 150
Audiologic assessment, 158
Auditory agnosia, 86, 87
  causes of, 89
Auditory cortex, 12
  lesions of, 88
Auditory discrimination disorders, 86–877
  causes of, 89
  representative quantitative and qualitative measure of, 180
Auditory information pathways, 24, 85, *86*
Auditory memory system, 119
Auditory nerve, 85
  dysfunction of, 89
Auditory system, 76. *See also* Deafness; Ears; Hearing.
  disorders of, 86–87

Auditory system *(cont.)*
causes of, 87–89
diagnosis of, 89
neuroanatomy of, 85
Auditory-linguistic dyslexia, 116–117
Auditory-verbal memory, 68
Autism, infantile, 148
Automatisms, 56
psychomotor, 55*t*
Autonomic nervous system, 4, 18–19
organs of, *20*
Axon, 4

Babinski reflex, 17
Babinski sign, 17
Basal ganglia, 9, 15, 99
Behavior
emotional
biological conditions associated with, 144*t*
chemical basis of, 142
neuroanatomical basis of, 140–141
psychotic, 149–150
psychomotor seizures and, 56*t*
sexual, 147
violent, 145, 146
Behavior abnormalities, 14, 139
chemical imbalance and, 146–147
developmental, 147–148
diagnosis of, 150–152
disruptive, 150
with epileptic seizures, 55, 57–58
neuroanatomical dysfunction and, 143–146
with split-brain surgery, 23–24
Bilateral mirror movement, 105
Binocular vision, 79–80
Blind spots, 80, 83
Blindness, 79. *See also* Visual disorders.
half-field, 83
pure word, 113
Body posture control, 101–102
Body schema disorders, 90, 94–97
representative quantitative and qualitative measure of, 181–182
Bordmann's system, *11*
Brain, 3. *See also specific areas of.*
afferent pathways to, 24–25
damage to
in adult, 29–31
associated with reading disorders, 112–113
dysfunction of, 26–27
age and, 28
causes of, in children and adults, 30*t*, 31
in children, 29–31
definition of, 26–27
features of, 27–28
individual factors in, 28
life circumstances and, 28
minimal, 150
signs of, 27
spatial acalculia with, 133
features of, neonatal and adult, 29
hemispheric specialization of. *See* Cerebral hemispheres.
insult to
characteristics of, 27–28
in mature vs. immature brain, 28–29
linguistic activity of, 35–36
parts of, 9–17
plasticity of, 28–29
tumors of, 24
writing skills and, 123–124
Brain stem, 3, 16, 99, 101
Brain-behavior research, 122–123, 153
Broca's aphasia, 38–39, 49
Broca's area, 114
Brodmann's system, 10

Calculation ability, 136. *See also* Arithmetic competence; Arithmetic disorders; Arithmetic subskills; Numbers.
impaired, 115–116
Carbamazepine, 60
Catecholamines, 142
Cell differentiation, 6
Central nervous system, 3
brain in, 9–17
critical growth period, 28
febrile illness and, 59
muscular activity and, 99
spinal cord in, 17
types of cell in, 8
Central sulcus, 9
Cerebellum, 3, 9, 17, 99
Cerebral cortex, 9, 99
anterior
higher association areas of, 14
motor areas of, 13–14
deep structures of, 3, 14–17
demarcations and lobes of, *10*
emotion and, 141
posterior, 10–12
higher association areas of, 12–13
sensory areas of, 12
sensory pathways in, 141
Cerebral hemispheres, 9
handedness and, 32
lateralization of, 19–21, 71
development of, 21–22
dysfunction of, 145–146
evidence for, 21
interhemispheric communication with, 23–24
ipsilateral and contralateral cortical representation in, 24–25
Cerebrospinal fluid, 9
Cerebrum, 3. *See also* Cerebral cortex; Cerebral hemispheres.

anterior cerebral cortex of, 13–14
deep structures of, 3, 14–17
functional regions of, 10–13
hemispheric specialization in. *See* Cerebral hemispheres, lateralization of.
higher association areas of, 12–13
interhemispheric communication in, 23–24
sensory areas of, 12
structural regions of, 9–10
Childhood seizure disorders, 58–59
diagnosis of, 59–60
etiology of, 59
psychologist's role in, 60–62
treatment of, 60
Children. *See also* Neonates.
brain dysfunction in, 29–31, 30*t*
emotional disorders in, 148–150
intellect of, vs. adult, 31
language of, 43–44
memory disorders in, 73
seizure disorders in, 58–62
Children's Apperception Test (CAT), 155
Circumlocutions, 38
Clinical observation guidelines, 173–174
CNS. *See* Central nervous system.
Cochlea, 85
Cochlear nerve destruction, 89
Cognitive function. *See also* Arithmetic competence; Language; Reading; Speech; Writing.
critical period for, 28
deficits in, 14
Colliculus, inferior, 85
Color agnosia, 81
Color vision, 77
Commissural disconnection syndrome, 24
Commissural fibers, 9
damage to, 115
Commissures, 23, *24*
Commissurotomy, 23–24
cerebral lateralization evidence from, 21
Communication, prelinguistic, 41. *See also* Language; Speech; Reading; Writing.
Comprehension, 36–37
aphasia of, 38–39
assessment of, 120
impaired, 125
of numerical concepts, 132
in reading process, 119
Comprehension-phonological syndrome, 44
Comprehensive psychological evaluation, 153–158
Computerized transaxial tomography, 157
Conduct disorder, 150
Conduction aphasia, 39
Conductive deafness, 86–87
causes of, 88
Cones, 77
Confabulation, 72
Conversational speech aphasias, 36
Coordination, 102
disorders of, 104, 106–107
Cornea, 77
Corpus callosum, damage to, 113, 115
Corti, 85
Cortical association fiber, damage to, 115
Cortical development stages, *30*
Cortical dysfunction, 82
in auditory disturbances, 88
blindness with, 83
in muscle tone disorders, 106
with touch disorders, 93
Corticospinal tracts, *100*, 101
of extrapyramidal pathways, *102*
Counting ability, 135
calculation abilities and, 136
Cranial nerves, 3, 18
eye movements and, 82
functions of, 19*t*
Critical periods, 28
Cultural-familial retardation, 33

Deafness, 86–87
causes of, 88–89
pure word, 87, 125
causes of, 89
Decoding, 35
in reading process, 118–119
skills, assessment of, 119–120
Deep phonological dyslexia, 117
Deep tendon reflexes, 17
Déjà vu, 54
Dendrites, 4
Depression, 145, 148–149
in conduct disorder, 150
with endocrine alteration, 146
Developmental behavioral disorders, pervasive, 147–148
Developmental handicap, 32
Dichotic listening
auditory pathways in, *23*
technique of, 21
Diencephalon, 9, 14–15
Dilantin, 60
Disconnection syndrome, 115
Discriminative function defect, 12
Disorientation, right-left, 95–96
Disruptive behavioral disorders, 150. *See also* Behavioral abnormalities; Hyperkinesis syndrome.
Dopamine, 8
Dopaminergic receptor blockage, 107
Double simultaneous discrimination disorder, 93
Down's syndrome, 33
DTR. *See* Deep tendon reflexes.
Dyscalculia, 133–135
Dyseidetic spelling, 127
Dysfluency, 49

Dysgraphia, 124, 126
  errors common in, 126–127
Dyslexia, 114–115, 116
  neurolinguistic subtypes of, 117
  neuropsychological subtypes of, 116–117
Dysorthographia, 124
Dysphasia, 43
Dysphonetic spelling, 126–127
Dyspraxias, 105–106

Ears. *See also* Auditory discrimination disorders; Auditory system; Deafness; Hearing.
  dysfunctions of, 86
  structures of, 85
Echolalia, 39
Efferent muscles, 3
Efferent nerve fibers, 8
Efferent pathways, 25
Electroencephalography, 157
Emotion
  biological basis of, 139–143
  chemical basis of, 142–143
  neuroanatomical basis of, 140–142
  in psychological evaluation, 154–155
Emotional behavior
  biological conditions associated with, 144*t*
  chemical basis of, 142
  neuroanatomical basis of, 140–141
Emotional disorders, 139
  chemical imbalance and, 146–147
  of childhood, 148–150
  diagnosis of, 150–152
  neuroanatomical dysfunction and, 143–146
  vs. seizure disorders, 57
Encephalitis, herpes simplex, 145
Encoding, 35
Endbrain, 9
Endocrine system, 141–142, 146
Endorphins, 147
Epileptic personality, 57–58
Epileptic seizure disorders, 51–52. *See also* Seizure disorders; Seizures.
  classification of, 52*t*
  definition of, 52
  diagnosis of, 59–60
  emotional features of, 145
  intellectual functioning and, 58
  personality and, 57–58
  spread of bioelectrical activity associated with, *53*
  treatment of, 60
  types of
    absence, 56
    complex partial, 54–55
    generalized, 56–57
    simple partial, 53–54
    simple partial that secondarily generalize, 55
    tonic-clonic, 56–57
Epinephrine, 8
Episodic disorders, 51–65
Episodic memory, 69
Equilibrium, control of, 17
Expressive language disturbance, 116
Expressive syndrome, severe, 44
Extracranial headaches, 63
Extrapyramidal motor system, 101–103
Eye. *See also* Blindness; Visual system.
  movements of
    impaired, 116
    involuntary, 79–80, 82
    voluntary, 82–83
  structures of, 77
Eyedness, 32

Farsightedness, 79
Febrile seizures, 59
Feedback pathways, 141
Fine motor coordination disorders, 106–107
Fine motor disturbances, 104
Finger agnosia, 94–95
Finger counting errors, 134
Fluency disorders, 49
Focal seizures, 53–55
Forced thinking, 54
Forebrain, 9–15
Forgetting, 69, 70
Frontal lobe syndrome, 143
Frontal lobes, 9, 101
  arithmetic competence and, 132
  damage to, writing disorders and, 125
  dysfunction in, 116, 143
  emotion and, 140
  emotional/behavioral disorders and, 143
  writing skills and, 123

Generic memory, 69
Geniculate nucleus, lateral, 78
Gerstmann syndrome, 97
Gilles de la Tourette's syndrome, 105
Glial cells, 8
Global aphasia, 39
Golgi cells, 8
Grammar, 128
  acquisition of, 41, 42
Grand mal seizure, 56–57
Graphomotor functions, 123. *See also* Writing; Writing disorders.
  deterioration of, 125
Gray matter, 8
Gross motor coordination disorders, 106
Gross motor disturbances, 104
Gyrus(i), 9. *See also specific gyri.*

Hallucination, olfactory, 54
Hand, right, regions controlling movement of, *108*
Handedness, 31–32
Handwriting, illegible, 127
Haptic imperception, 93
Headaches
  continuous and acute, 63
  diagnosis of, 63
  etiology of, 63
  intermittent and recurrent, 62–63
  psychologist's role with, 64–65
  treatment of, 64
  types of, 62–63
Hearing. *See also* Auditory system; Deafness; Ears.
  disorders of, 86–89
  neuroanatomical basis of, 85
Hemianopia, 80
Hemiparesis, 106
Herpes simplex encephalitis, 145
Heschl's gyrus, 85
Hindbrain, 9, 16–17
Hippocampus, 71
Homunculus
  motor, 13, *14*, 101
  sensory, *13, 92*
Hormones, 142, 146
House-Tree-Person test (H-T-P), 155
Hyperactive child syndrome, 150
Hyperkinesis syndrome, 150
Hyperopia, 79
Hypertonia, 104
  causes of, 106
Hypothalamotomy, 145
Hypothalamus, 14, 15
  dysfunction of, 145
  emotion and, 141, 142
Hypotonia, 104
  causes of, 106

Ideational dyspraxia, 106
Ideomotor dyspraxia, 106
Impulsivity, 145
Infantile autism, 148
Intellect
  of adults vs. children, 31
  epilepsy and, 58
Intelligence quotient (IQ), 32
Intention tremors, 105
Interbrain, 9, 14–15
Interhemispheric commissures, 23
Interictal behavioral alterations, 57–58
Interictal interval, 52
Interneuronal communication, *6*, 7–8
Interpersonal relationships, language acquisition and, 40–41
Intraictal period, 52
Invariant tic, 105
Involuntary movements, abnormal, 104–105, 107
Involuntary muscles, 4

Jamais vu, 54

Kluver-Bucy syndrome, 145

Language. *See also* Alexia; Dyslexia; Reading; Speech; Writing.
  acquisition of, 40
    timetable for, 41–43
  adult disorders of, 36
    classification of, 36–39
  assessment of competence in, 46–47
  critical period for learning of, 28
  decoding and encoding of, 35
  detection of, 34
  developmental requirements of, 40–41
  discrimination of, 34
  disorders of, 34–50
    acquired, 43
    behavioral and emotional characteristics of, 47*t*
    of childhood, 43–44
    developmental, 43–45
    diagnosis of, 45–47
    emotional/behavioral disorders and, 143
    expressive, 116
    receptive, 44, 116, 124–125
    writing disorders with, 122–123
  impaired comprehension of, 125
  interpretation of, 34
  neuroanatomical basis of, 34–36
  nuances of, 40
  oral, 42–43
  reception of, 34
  representative quantitative and qualitative measure of, 176
  skills of
    numerical word problem solving and, 136
    in reading comprehension, 119
  subskills of, 46–47
  written, 43
Language-related speech disorders, 48
Left-handedness, 32
Lemniscal pathways, *91*
  lateral, 85
Lemniscal system, 91–92
  dysfunction of, 94
Lens, 77
Letter rotation/inversion, 127
Letter reversal, 127
Letter substitution/omissions, 127
Letter-sound associations, 118, 119
  disorder of, 117
Limbic circuit, 71

Limbic system, 15
  dysfunction of, 143–145, 149, 150
  emotion and, 140, 141
  emotional/behavioral disorders and, 143–145
  structures of, *72, 142*
Linguistic activity, 35–36
Linguistic errors, 126
  in arithmetic disorders, 135
Listening, dichotic
  auditory pathways in, *23*
  technique of, 21
Locomotor development, 109, 110
Longitudinal sulcus, 9
Long-term memory
  processes of, 69–70
  store of, 70–71
  varieties of, 69
Luminal, 60

Macroscopia, 54
Maladaptive reaction, 149
Mammillary bodies, 15, 71
Manic-depression, 146, 149
Manipulation skills, development of, 109–110
Medulla, 9, 16
Memory. *See also* Memory disorders.
  arithmetic competence and, 132
  arithmetic subskills and, 137
  assessment of functions of, 73–74
  epileptic seizures and, 54
  failure of. *See* Amnesia; Forgetting.
  interference with, 70
  neuroanatomical basis of, 71
  processes of, 67
  in reading process, 119
  representative quantitative and qualitative measure of, 177
  search, 70
  structure of, 66
  study of, 66–67
  subcortical focus of, 71
  systems of
    interaction of, 70–71
    long-term, 69–70
    sensory buffer, 67–68
    short-term, 68–69
  tests of, 73–74
  trace, 69–70
    decay of, 70
  tricks for, 70
  visual-spatial, 119
Memory disorders
  assessment of, 73–74
  in children, 73
  historical background of, 66–67
  types of, 71–73
Meninges, 9
Mental deficiency, 32
Mental retardation, 32–33
  categories of, 32
  classification of, 33
  factors in, 32–33
Mesencephalon, 9, 16
Metamorphosia, 54
Microscopia, 54
Midbrain, 9, 16
Migraine, 63. *See also* Headaches.
Miller's magic number, 68
Mirror movement, 105
Mirror writing, 127
Mnemonics, 70
Mood disorders, 148–149. *See also* Depression; Manic-depression.
Motor cortex, 13–14
  dysfunction of, 48
Motor discoordination dyslexia, 117
Motor disorders, 99, 103–104
  of abnormal movements, 104–105
  causes of, 106–108
  with cerebellum dysfunction, 17
  classifications of, 103–104
  of coordination, 104, 117
  diagnosis of, 110
  of learned skilled motor acts, 105–106
  of tone and strength, 104
  representative quantitative and qualitative measure of, 183–184
  writing disorders with, 122
Motor functions
  in emotional/behavioral evaluation, 151
  neuroanatomical basis of, 99–103
  voluntary, 100–101
Motor homunculus, 13, *14*, 101
Motor neurons
  lower, 100–101
  pathways of, 3
  upper, 100–101, 103
Motor perseveration, 143
Motor skills
  acquisition timetable for, 108–110
  critical period for, 28
Motor system
  development of, 108–110
  dysfunction of, 48
Movement
  abnormal associated, 105
    causes of, 107
  abnormal involuntary, 104–105
    causes of, 107
  disorders of learned skilled, 105–106
    causes of, 108
Multiple tic syndrome, 105
Muscle strength disorders, 104
  causes of, 106
Muscle tone disorders, 104
  causes of, 106

Muscles. *See also* Motor disorders; Motor functions.
  control of, 99
  relaxation of, 103
Musculoskeletal system, 76
Myelin sheaths, 5
  formation of, 8
Myelination, 5
Myopia, 79

Naming, 37
  impaired, 116
Nearsightedness, 79
Neonates. *See also* Children.
  brain features of, 29
  seizure disorders in, 58–59
Nerve deafness, 87
  causes of, 88–89
Nerve(s). *See also* Neurons; *specific nerves*.
  afferent and efferent, 17
  fibers of, 4–5
    types of, 8–9
  impulses, 4, 7–8
  peripheral, 3
Nervous system. *See also* Autonomic nervous system; Central nervous system; Parasympathetic nervous system; Periphral nervous system; Somatic nervous system; Sympathetic nervous system.
  cerebral organization in, 19–25
  critical periods in development of, 28
  neurons in, 4–9
  organization of, 3–4
Neural tube, 9
Neurochemical brain pathway disturbance, 107
Neuroglia, 8
Neurolinguistic language disorders, 44–45
Neurology assessment, 157
Neuromuscular endings, 3
Neuronal circuit, 7–8
Neurons, 4–5. *See also* Nerve(s).
  growth and development of, 6–7
  interneuronal communication of, 7–8
  nerve fiber types in, 8–9
  types of, 8
Neuropeptides, 142, 147
Neuropsychological function, 156
  in comprehensive psychological evaluation, 157*t*
  disorders of, 1
  of language, 44
Neuropsychology, developmental, 29–31
Neurotransmitters
  disordered metabolism of, 150
  emotion and, 142, 146
  release of, 8
Norepinephrine, 8
Numbers. *See also* Arithmetic competence; Calculation ability.
  agraphia for, 133
  comprehension of, 135
    calculation abilities and, 136
    errors in, 134
  concept errors of, 134
  inversions/rotations of, 134
  misalignment errors of, 134
  sequence errors of, 134
  skills of, practical, 137
Numerical concepts, 132
Numerical word problem solving, 136
Nystagmus, 80, 82

Object angosia, 81
Occipital lobe, 9, 78
  arithmetic competence and, 132
  damage to, 113
  lesion in, 115
  in reading process, 114
Ocular dysmetria, 8, 83
Ocular dyspraxia, 80, 83
Ocular motility disorders, 79–80
  causes of, 82–83
Olfactory hallucinations, 54
Olfactory nerve replacement, 6
Ophthalmologic assessment, 158
Optic chiasm, 78
Optic nerve, 77–78
  dysfunction of, 83
Oromotor apraxia, 117
Overwriting, 125

Paralysis, 104
  causes of, 106
Paraparesis, 106
Paraphasias, 38, 39, 125
Parasympathetic nervous system, 4, 18–19
Parent (guardian) interview
  in headache treatment, 64
  in language skills assessment, 46
  in psychological evaluation, 154
  for seizure disorders, 61
Paresis, 104
  causes of, 106
Parietal cortex, 9, 92
  arithmetic competence and, 132
  dysfunction of, 95–97
    with apraxic agraphia, 126
    with reading-writing disorder, 116
  writing skills and, 123
Pastel classic signs, 27
Pathological handedness, 32
Patient history sample, 168–169
Peripheral nerves, 3
  dysfunction of, 48

Peripheral nervous system, 3, 17–18, 17–19
  in muscular activity control, 99
  nerve fibers in, 4–5
Peripheral visual field restriction, 83
Perseveration, 106, 127
  causes of, 108
  errors, 135
Personality disorders, 149
  epilepsy and, 57–58
Personality tests, 155
Petit mal seizures, 54*t*
Phenobarbital, 60
Phenothiazines, side effects of, 107
Phenylketonuria, 33
Phenytoin, 60
Phonemes. *See* Speech sounds.
Phonological dyslexia, 117
Phonological-syntactical syndrome, 45
Phonology, acquisition of, 41
Pineal gland, 15
Pituitary gland, 15
PNS. *See* Peripheral nervous system.
Pons, 9, 16
Postcentral gyrus dysfunction, 93–94
Postictal period, 52
Postsynaptic membranes, 7–8
Postural tremors, 104–105, 107
Posture, body, control of, 101–102
Precentral cortex, 140
Precentral gyrus, 13, 101
Prefrontal lobe, 124
Prelinguistic communication, 41
Premenstrual disorders, 146
Premotor cortex, 13–14
Prenatal nervous system, critical periods in, 28
Presynaptic membranes, 7, 8
Problem solving ability, 136
Progressive lateralization theory, 22
Projection fibers, 8
Proprioceptors, 103
Prosody, 146
  of speech, 145
    disorders of, 49
Prospagnosia, 81
Pseudoepileptic seizures, 57*t*
Psychiatric assessment, 158
Psychological evaluation, 153
  emotional factors in, 154–155
  neuropsychological factors in, 156
  prescriptive treatment recommendations of, 158
  recommendations for, 156–158
  social factors in, 153–154
Psychologist
  in headache treatment, 64–65
  in seizure disorders, 60–62
Psychomotor agitation, 149
Psychomotor automatisms, 55*t*
Psychomotor retardation, 143
Psychomotor seizures vs. psychotic behavior, 56*t*
Psychosis, secondary, 146
Psychotic behavior, 149–150
  psychomotor seizures and, 56*t*
Pyramidal motor system, 100–101, 103
  dysfunction of, 107

Quadriparesis, 106

Ranvier, nodes of, 5
RAS. *See* Reticular activating system.
Reading, 37. *See also* Reading disorders; Writing.
  competence and skills of, 119–120
  comprehension in, 119
  decoding steps of, 118–119
  learning of, 43
  neuroanatomical basis of, 114
  process of, 118–119
  representative quantitative and qualitative measure of, 185–186
  subskills of
    assessment of, 119–120
    representative quantitative and qualitative measure of, 187–190
  tests for, 119–120
Reading disorders
  clinical syndromes of, 114–118
  diagnosis of, 118–119
  historical background of, 112–114
  with writing disturbance, 113
Recent memory, 69
Receptive language disturbance, 116
Reflexes
  deep, 17
  development of, 109–110
  spinal, 17
  superficial, 17
Remembering, stages of, 67
Remote memory, 69
Repetition, 37
  impaired, 39
Retardation
  cultural-familial, 33
  mental, 32–33
  psychomotor, 143
Reticular activating system, 16, 55
  emotion and, 140–141
Reticular formation, ascending, 85
Retina, 77
Retrograde amnesia, 72
Right hand, regions controlling movement of, *108*
Right-left disorientation, 95–96
Rigidity, causes of, 106
Rods, 77
Rooting reflex, 109
Rorschach test, 155

Schema disorders, body, 90, 94–97
  representative quantitative and qualitative measure of, 181–182
Schizophrenia, 145, 149–150
  etiology of subtypes of, 146*t*
School report
  in language skills assessment, 46–47
  in psychological evaluation, 155
  sample of, 170–172
  for seizure disorders, 61
Scotoma, central, 83
Seizure disorders. *See also* Epileptic seizure disorders.
  diagnosis of, 59–60
  etiology of, 59
  febrile, 59
  in infancy and childhood, 58–62
  neonatal, 58–59
  psychologist's role with, 60–62
  treatment of, 60
Seizures, 59
  absence, 56
  febrile, 59
  focal, 53–55
  grand mal, 56–57
  petit mal, 54*t*
  pseudoepileptic, 57*t*
  psychomotor, vs. psychotic behavior, 56*t*
  visual disorders with, 54
Selective arousal and attention system, 140–141, 150
  emotional/behavioral disorders and, 143
Semantic-pragmatic syndrome, 44
Semantics, 128
  acquisition of, 41
Sensory areas, 12
  emotion and, 140
  emotional/behavioral disorders and, 143
Sensory buffer, 67–68, 70
Sensory feedback, 103
Sensory homunculus, *13, 92*
Sensory information
  emotion and, 140–141
  pathways of, 3, 17, 140–141
  processing of, 10
  storage of, 68
Sensory projection dysfunction, 143
Sensory receptors, 3
Sensory register, 68
Sensory/perceptual disorders, 76–97. *See also specific disorders; specific senses.*
Sequencing abilities, 132
Serotonin, 142
Severe expressive syndrome, 44
Sexual behavior, 147
Short-term memory, 68–69
  register of, 70
Sidedness, 32
Simultanagnosia, 81
Skin structures, 90–91
Social development, 153–154
Social relationships, 28
Soft signs, 27
Soma, 4
Somatic nervous system, 3
Somatosensory acuity, 118
Somatosensory cortex, 12
  afferent pathways to, 24
Somatosensory discrimination, 128
Somatosensory information pathways, 25
  central, 93
Somatosensory processing, 93
Somatosensory receptors, 103
Somatosensory system, 76, 89–90. *See also* Touch.
  disorders of, 92–93
    causes of, 93–94
    diagnosis of, 94
  neuroanatomy of, 90–92
Sound blending disorder, 117
Sound discrimination disturbances. *See* Auditory discrimination disorders.
Sound interpretation, 12
Sound-letter associations, 128
Sound-letter conversion, 123
Spasticity, 106
Spatial agraphia, 125–126
Spatial disorganization, 127
  and arithmetic disorders, 134
Speech. *See also* Language; Speech sounds.
  agrammatical, 125
  articulation of, 38
  automatic, 48
  conversational, 36
  discrimination disturbance of, 125
  disorders of, 47–50
  errors of, 38
  first words of, 41–42
  impaired fluency of, 39
  neuroanatomical basis of, 47–48
  prosody of, 145
  reception and discrimination of, 123
  representative quantitative and qualitative measure of, 176
Speech sounds
  acquisition of, 41
  dysfunction of discrimination of, 89
  segmenting of, 128
Speech/language pathologic assessment, 158
Spelling
  defective written, 127
  disturbances of, 125–126
  dyseidetic, 127
  dysphonetic, 126–127
  oral, 127
  performance, 120
Spinal cord, 3, 17, 99
Spinal nerves, 18

Spinal reflexes, 17
Spinothalamic system, 91
Split-brain effect, *22*
Split-brain surgery, 21, 23–24
Status epilepticus, 52
Strabismus, 80, 82
Subcortical auditory pathway dysfunctions, 88
Sulcus(i), 9
Surface phonological dyslexia, 117
Syllable inversion, 127
Syllable substitution/omissions, 127
Sylvian fissure, 9
Sympathetic nervous system, 4, 18–19
Synapses, 4
  interneuronal communication at, 7–8
Syntax, 128
  acquisition of, 41

Tactile localization disorder, 93
Tactile somatosensory system. *See* Touch.
Tactile stimulation, 93
  impaired interpretation of, 12
Tay-Sachs disease, 33
Tegretol, 60
Telegraphic writing, 125
Telencephalon, 9
Temporal lobe, 9
  arithmetic competence and, 132
  dysfunction in, 116
  writing skills and, 123
Test distributors and publishers, 167
Thalamus, 14, 15, 78
  emotion and, 141
Thematic Apperception Test (TAT), 155
Thought blocking, 54
Tics, 105
  causes of, 107
Tomography, computerized transaxial, 157
Tonic-clonic seizures, 55, 56–57
Topographical orientation defect, 81
Touch
  disorders of, 92–93
    causes of, 93–94
    diagnosis of, 94
  neuroanatomical basis of, 90–92
  representative quantitative and qualitative measure of, 181
Transcortical mixed aphasia, 39
Transcortical motor aphasia, 39
Transcortical sensory aphasia, 39
Transient tic syndrome, 105
Transverse temporal gyrus, 85
Tremors, 104–105
  postural, 107
Tumors, brain, 24
Two-point discrimination disorder, 93

Unilateral mirror movement, 105
Unilateral visual neglect, 81

Verbal agnosia, 89
  auditory, 45, 87
Verbal apraxia, 49
Verbal intelligence tests, 129
Vestibular nuclei, 103
Violent behavior, 145, 146
Visceral organs, 76
Vision. *See also* Blindness; Visual cortex; Visual disorders; Visual system; *specific disorders of.*
  neuroanatomical basis of, 77–78
Visual acuity, disorders of, 79
  causes of, 82
Visual agnosia, 80–81, 116
Visual cortex, 12
  damage to, 113
Visual discrimination, 128
  disorder of, 80
Visual disorders. *See also* Blindness.
  representative quantitative and qualitative measure of, 178–179
  constructive, 81
    causes of, 83
  with seizures, 54
Visual field, defects of, 80, *84*
  causes of, 83
Visual information
  pathways of, 24, 77–78
    critical growth period for, 28
  processing disorders of, 80–81, 83
  transmission of, 81
Visual neglect, unilateral, 81
Visual perceptual/recognition disorders, 80–81
  causes of, 83
Visual receptors, 103
Visual spatial memory functions, 73
Visual system, 76
  disorders of, 78–81
    causes of, 81–83
    diagnosis of, 83
    unilateral, 81–82
  neuroanatomy of, 77–78
Visual-auditory association, 118
Visual-kinesthetic information, 123
Visual-spatial functions
  arithmetic competence and, 132
  disorders of, 13, 81
    acalculia with, 133
    causes of, 83
  writing disturbances and, 123
Visual-spatial memory, 119
Visual-spatial perceptual dyslexia, 117
Vocabulary acquisition, 41–42
Voice disorders, 49
Voluntary muscles, 3

Wernicke's aphasia, 37–38
Wernicke's area, 114
White matter, 8
WISC-R Coding subtest, 61
Word blindness, pure, 113
Word deafness, pure, 87, 125
  causes of, 89
Word substitution/omissions, 125, 127
Word-label associations, 118
Word-visual image conversion, 123
Work pattern, inappropriate, 134–135
Writing, 37. *See also* Writing disorders.
  competence of
    assessment of, 128–130
    representative quantitative and qualitative measure of, 191
  learning of, 43
  mirror, 127
  neuroanatomical basis of, 123–124
  process of, 127–129
  subskills of
    assessment of, 128–130
    representative quantitative and qualitative measure of, 192–195
  telegraphic, 125
  testing of, 129
Writing disorders, 38
  clinical syndromes of, 124–127
  diagnosis of, 127–130
  errors made with, 126*t*
  historical background on, 122–123
  with reading disorders, 113